Myrtle B. Findley's

Real Food

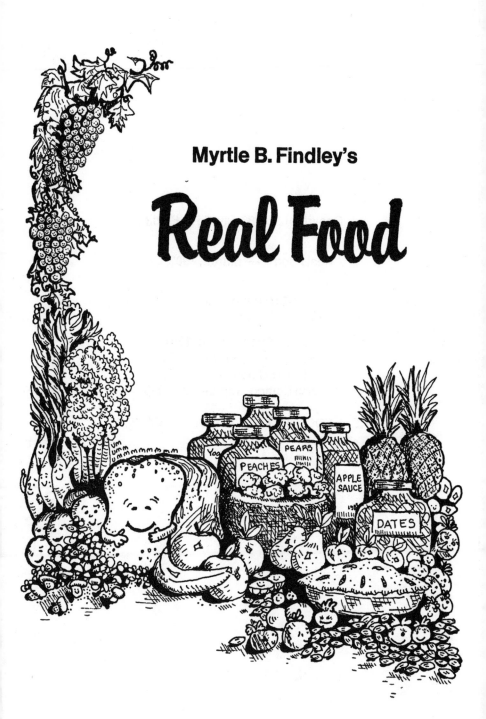

Real Food™ — March, 1983, CA

ISBN: 0-9611550-0-0

First Edition, March, 1981
Second Edition, July, 1981
Third Edition, May, 1982
Fourth Edition, September, 1983

REAL FOOD, P.O. Box 721, Colfax, CA 95713

MYRTLE B. FINDLEY'S

Real Food

... a simple natural, unrefined food
as is grown and harvested from
the garden, orchard, or field, or as found in
many grocery markets

... a food which is then prepared without
the use of grease, oil, or refined foods

... a food kept free of unnecessary additives
or unnecessary deletions

... an easy method of building and maintaining
a diet with 15% to 20% fat from only natural
and nutritious sources

... This is Real Food.

Front cover design by my son, Robert Mark Findley

DEDICATION

This book is dedicated to my husband, Bob. I thank him for saying "yes" several years ago when I asked him to join me in a diet without refined foods or fats. Now, we both share in the delight of full true flavors from fruits, vegetables, all grain dishes, breads, and YES . . . desserts!

Myrtle B. Findley

WHY REAL FOOD?

A modification in the diet has been shown to prevent and aid in treatment of all degenerative diseases: strokes, hardening of the arteries, hypertension, cancer, diabetes, hypoglycemia, kidney stones, gout, arthritis, and obesity.

Modifying the diet strikes at the source of the problem and affects a LONG-TERM restorative process. Other means used only cover up symptoms while the underlying disease condition continues.

Many magazine, TV, and news articles today speak of the need to use less fats and protein in our American diets. We are now told fats should compose only 15 to 20% of the diet. The average American diet consists of 40 to 45%. Besides fats, many other changes need to made in our diets.

REAL FOOD is designed to help those interested in making this change to get to it. Real Food encourages reading and research. Resources are available. DIG IN!

ALLERGIC?

Can't eat wheat? or oats? or barley? or rice?
Find recipes just for you in REAL FOOD.

Can't eat sugar? Can't eat raisins or dates?
Find a sweetener just for you in REAL FOOD.

Many recipes adjust for individual allergies.

What is "Real Food" all about?

. . . Cook it in your own kitchen . . .

REAL FOOD recipes were first prepared so patients leaving a live-in health center could continue on a therapeutic diet at home by having recipes to follow and use in their own kitchen.

. . . Shop mainly in Produce sections of grocery markets . . .

REAL FOOD cookbook emphasizes the use of fresh fruits, fresh vegetables, fresh whole grains, seeds, legumes, and most all of the unprocessed harvest as grown. Simply wash and clean. This food can then be kitchen-prepared using the complete whole produce and not eliminating and discarding parts which will provide valuable elements for healing and health of the body.

. . . Be selective in shopping . . .

REAL FOOD cookbook de-emphasizes the use of commercially packaged foods as found on the shelves of most grocery stores. Read labels in the canned, packaged, and processed departments of the market. These foods have fats, sugars, and salts added in the packaging and processing, as well as eliminating and destroying parts of the original fruit, vegetable, grain, nut, seed, or legume.

. . . DO IT YOURSELF:

With a home food processor:
Many soft grains, dried fruits, or legumes and some rolled grains can be easily ground or broken for use in Real Food recipes.

With a home food blender:
All rolled grains and many whole softer grains or legumes may be made into coarse flours for use in Real Food recipes.

With a home mill:
— Many types of beans, legumes, etc.
— All types of rice
— All types of corn
— All types of grains
— Some seeds can be ground very fine to be used in Real Food recipes.

Note: Read mill instructions for details.

ASK FOR THESE IN YOUR NATURAL GROCERY MARKET . . .

Whole Grains	Cracked Grains	Rolled Grains
Oats*	Wheat	Oats
Wheat	Rye	Wheat
Tricale	Millet	Barley
Barley*	Oats	Rye
Rye	Buckwheat	
Millet*	Corn	
Buckwheat	Tricale	
Amaranth*		
Rice*	**Ground or Flour Grains**	
	Corn	Oats
Puffed Grains	Rye	Barley
Rice	Wheat	Rice
Wheat	Buckwheat	Millet
	Tricale	Amaranth

Designates softer type grains

Baked or Dextrinized

Bulgar	Rice
Wheat	Barley
Rye	Tricale

ASK FOR THESE IN YOUR REGULAR GROCERY MARKETS . . .

Fruits and berries	Vegetables:
Sprouts	*Above and below ground*
Seeds	Fat-, sugar-free crackers
Sprouted grain breads	Fat-, sugar-free breads

A REAL FOOD KITCHEN/PANTRY WILL NEED:

powdered arrowroot
baking yeast
powdered and flakes of onion
powdered and flakes of garlic
powdered and flakes of leaves of herbs
unsweetened grated or shredded coconut
canned fruits in natural juices (or home canned)
canned WHOLE tomatoes (less additives)
fresh lemons
fresh fruits and vegetables as they come in season

ALL sorts of grains as listed and in all forms: whole, rolled,
    cracked, ground

ALL sorts of legumes and ALL kinds of beans.
    Store in large glass jars with lids for easy viewing.

Buy in bulk: dried dates, currants, raisins, fruits.
Buy on sale: peel and freeze . . . ripe bananas.

whole grain (various types) pastas

a food blender

a food processor (if possible)

a food freezer

room for storage in refrigerator

other equipment as desired for home processing and
    convenience, such as a dehydrator, a grain
    mill, nut grinder, a microwave oven

STEPS TOWARD A REAL FOOD KITCHEN (allow up to 2 years)

Step 1. Slowly eliminate foods from your pantry which are not REAL FOOD.

Step 2. Learn to sauté and fry with small amounts of water instead of traditional grease, fats, and oils.

Step 3. Learn to eat all the fat/sugar free bread you want.
— Make or buy bread without fat or sugar.
— Look for sprouted grain breads; they are best!

Step 4. Learn to convert conventional recipes:
— Use water instead of milks or cream.
— Use Real Food pastes for sugars and honey.
— Simply OMIT shortening, margarines, and oils!
— Re-think a recipe in terms of:
  extenders   binders   flavoring   nutrition

Step 5. — Use ripe fruits as natural sweeteners instead of the highly refined sugar beets, sugar canes, honey or molasses.
— Use such items as arrowroot for sauces, glazes, frostings, creams . . . in place of butter.
— Make a cake without milk, sugar, fats, eggs or white flour.
— Make a pie crust without shortening or white flour.
— Discover grains, legumes, new foods!
— Work without dairy products at all!
— Learn to use nuts sparingly.
— Avoid vitamin "D" products.

Step 6. Learn to make a meal with single food items; or use foods from same family; then skip that family for several days. GOOD FOR ALLERGIES.
Curcurbitaceae, SQUASHES
Solanaceae
Leguminoseae
Rosaceae, STONE FRUITS
Dioscoreaceae
Umbelliferae, etc. . . . .

Step 7. Omit irritating spices such as cinnamon, nutmeg, ginger, pepper, vinegar, pickles . . . as well as baking powder, baking soda, and such. See glossary.

Step 8. READ ALL LABELS COMPLETELY and learn what is not listed, but is included in package.

Storage Suggestions

"I've got bugs in my cereal"

INSECTS Many natural Real Food items may be affected by insects, so care should be taken to keep cool and/or refrigerated. (Freezing helps kill infestations)

NEED HELP If rice, corn, grain or seeds become infested with insects: wash with cold water. Flood and pour off flying insects and larvae . . . clean well. Cook at once while still wet, or, most grains and seeds can be saved by careful drying in a warm slow oven and then refrigerate until used.

REFRIGERATOR A REAL FOOD kitchen uses the refrigerator in a new manner for storage of REAL FOOD.

Bags of grains need to be stored in the refrigerator. An additional shelf on the door makes a nice bin for bags of dried fruits, grains, or nuts. An additional shelf in the refrigerator makes additional storage for fresh fruits in season. Shelves need only be far enough apart to allow air circulation. A refrigerator could take 2 to 3 more shelves to store vegetables and fruits. i.e.: 15# of pitted Mejool dates in a large bag fits nicely in meat drawer of most refrigerators for immediate access.

Two Diets

or eating patterns are included in this REAL FOOD cookbook. A **Therapeutic Diet** and a **Maintenance Diet.** The Maintenance way is a suggested daily, year-around pattern for those in good health to maintain that health. The THERAPEUTIC LEVEL of diet is for those who wish to hasten regeneration of the body and bring about an accelerated healing pattern. It is recommended for those with a "problem". When the problem is overcome, then return to the Maintenance pattern. Real Food was written especially for those interested in a THERAPEUTIC LEVEL supplemented with Maintenance when desired.

... Therefore, all recipes at the THERAPEUTIC LEVEL will be marked with the code (t) to help quickly identify.

This REAL FOOD cookbook was written so a patient can enjoy a variety of foods, and desserts while staying on the Therapeutic healing diet. Let your body heal and regenerate itself ... and still enjoy eating food ... REAL FOOD!

A Therapeutic Diet

Use for a daily eating pattern to hasten relief of 'problem'.

This diet like this book is designed for those who need an immediate accelerated benefit to health. This is a very low fat diet therapy and is not expected to be adopted as a lifetime diet. Use for periods of one full year, six months, or less, until the "problem" is under control; then relax to the Maintenance Diet and periodically return. Frequent returning to A THERAPEUTIC DIET will prove rewarding.

ENJOY!
No Limits on

Fruits, vegetables, sprouts: cooked or raw.

All legumes.

All whole grains: cereals, desserts, breads, entrées, soups and salads.

Fat-free and sugar-free breads and crackers (read labels carefully).

All REAL FOOD recipes marked with (*t*) are acceptable.

ELIMINATE!

Natural fats of: avocado, olives, nuts, fish, poultry, eggs, raw milk, raw cream, yogurts, all diary products.

Oils, lards, shortening, margarines, hard cheeses, mayonnaise, and all foods containing such. All fried foods. Meat and all analogs (or imitations), as well as sugar, honey, pickles, vinegar, salts, alcohol, colas, soy and gluten products. All white flour and such highly processed flours. Coffee and tea. Generally ALL commercially processed and highly refined foods.

Read labels carefully.

ESTABLISH Patterns

Regular meals at least 4 hours apart, preferably 5 hours with NO between meal snacks to slow down digestion. DRINK only WATER between meals.

EXERCISE

and sunbathe as prescribed by a physician.

A Maintenance Diet

Use for a daily eating pattern to maintain good health, once re-established.

ENJOY *No Limits on*

    Fruits, vegetables, sprouts: cooked or raw.
    Dextrinized or plain whole grain berries
    All legumes
    Seeds
    Fat-, sugar-free sprouted grain breads
    REAL FOOD breads
    All REAL FOOD recipes

and these, but NOT every day!

Natural fats of: avocado, olives, nuts, fish, poultry, limited meats, eggs, (2-3 wk.) raw milk, raw cream, unsweetened yogurt, yogurt cultures, salt and very limited sugar or honey. (No recipes in REAL FOOD contain sugar or honey.)

ELIMINATE

Processed fats: hard cheeses, all oils (including cold pressed) margarines, salad dressings, and mayonnaise. Lards, shortenings, meats, all meat analogs (imitations), all greasy fried foods.

Vitamin "D" milk and such products (including ice cream and ice milks), white breads and all breads made with fats and sugars, oil/salted nuts and such, potato chips, crackers, coffee, tea, alcohol, colas, soy and gluten products.

Watch for hidden fats, sugars and salts in beverages, cold cereals, canned and frozen foods, gums, dressings, dry mixes, crackers, etc. Avoid commercially processed, highly refined, unnatural foods. Read all labels.

ESTABLISH Patterns

Enjoy regular meals 4 to 5 hours apart. No between meal snacks to slow digestion. Enjoy drinking only water between meals.

EXERCISE

and sunbathe as prescribed by physician.

PERMITTED

Raw Milk: Bring to 161°, cool, refrigerate, then limit to 12 oz. per day. Roast peanuts, cashews, etc., in oven. Discover: Soft cheese, such as Real Food cheeses, and other cheeses with only 1 gram fat per cup, such as nonfat yogurts, dry curds, hoop cheese. Also try Kefir and Neufchatel-type cheese. Experiment with various herbs for seasoning (see index).

IS THE CUPBOARD BARE?

LEGUMES:

Seeds in pods:
| Beans | Lentils | Peas |
| Chickpeas | Peanuts | Soybeans |

PEAS:

Whole sweet dried: good in casserole soups or as table vegetable

Split green: soups, casseroles, etc.
Split yellow: soups, casseroles, etc.

LENTILS:

Brown/green or yellow/red

Cooks quickly: for soups, casseroles
Sprouts easily

GARBANZO:

Tan/natural in color (Chickpeas)

Soak, clean and sort before cooking. Use in salads, casseroles, snacks, and main dishes. Sprouts easily.

BEANS:

Wash to remove small stones or dirt often found in beans. Soak overnight. Rinse. Cook slowly till skin peels and beans soften before adding salt and seasonings. Some sprout.

Great Northern	Pink	Black
Red Kidney	Lima	Mungs
Pinquinto	Soy	Fava
White Kidney	Pinto	Navy
White Marrowfat	Wing	Blackeye
Swedish Brown	and many, many more

MILLET:

Yellow, similar to corn and cornmeal. Use whole as cereal, ground in blender as a cream cereal, or whole stirred into bread batter or mixed into casseroles. Fairly mild and bland. Sprouts.

BUCKWHEAT:

Not a grain but a seed. Fairly strong flavor. Use as flour. Use as cereal, but best if mixed with corn, rice, or millet. High biologic value, rich in vitamins and minerals. Sprouts easily.

CORN:

Yellow corn and white corn

Field and sweet corn. Dried sweet corn good for snacking and chewing on hikes. Use for cereal, casseroles, soups, etc. Cracked corn, coarse cornmeal, fine cornmeal.
Soak for snacks.

RICE:

Natural rices: long grain, short grain, sweet rices, etc.

May be dextrinized for quick cooking, see pg. 34. Cook in pot with at least one inch of water covering. Slowly simmer and keep warm for one hour. Turn off heat and leave over warm burner or over double boiler to continue swelling and full cooking. No Stir to break texture.

BULGAR:

Pre-baked and broken grains of either wheat or rye:

Pour boiling water over: 2 parts water to 1 part grain. Cover and keep warm till tender. Use in salads or casseroles or plain as main dish.

AMARANTH:

Small Mustard seed size. New to market! Use as millet. Use for cereal, breads, casseroles, etc.

BEAN THREADS:

Spaghetti shaped threads made of bean flour; cooks translucent and absorbs flavor of dish it accompanies.

Available in Eastern specialty stores.

RICE STICKS:

Threads of rice. Soak in hot water and add to sautéed vegetables, etc.

Available in eastern specialty stores.

SHOP ETHNIC AND SPECIALTY GROCERY MARKETS

PREFACE

Breakfast Recipes

Breakfast Cereals

REAL FOOD DRY CEREAL MIX (Use as a staple snack)

HEAT AND LIGHTLY BROWN: **3 to 4 cups of rolled grains** such as barley, oats, rye, wheat, etc. . . . in 350° oven together with nuts.

SOAK: **Raisins, currants,** or any overly **dried fruits** until soft, then pat dry.

CUT: Fruits into small pieces. (Fruits such as figs, apricots, pears, apples, peaches, etc.)

COOK: a **couple raw apples** and blend with a few softened **dates or raisins** to sweeten and make about 1 c of applesauce in the food blender. Set aside to cool.

WHEN TOASTED:

Pour about 3 to 4 cups of the grains into a large mixing bowl. Add the chopped fruits, and such items as:

sunflower seeds to taste
wheat germ to taste
chopped **dates**
currants
coconut
nuts (omit for therapeutic level)

Pour the warm applesauce over the whole mixture just prepared and use hands to squeeze together and mix well. Leave some pieces in hunks.

HOT CEREALS (*t*)

Proportions in the following recipes vary depending on the particular type of grain used and the length of cooking (or reheating) time. Taste test!

WHOLE GRAIN BERRIES (Oats, Barley, Rye, Wheat, etc.)

4 c boiling water
1 c whole grain of choice

ADD grain to pot of boiling water. PLACE pot on medium-low heat and COOK slowly for 20 to 40 minutes.

Note: Best if soaked overnight before cooking or simmered in crockpot till ready to eat. Long, slow cooking enhances the flavor of whole grains! (Try cooking by the pound and refrigerate excess. Reheat in microwave or double boiler.)

GROUND GRAINS (whole grain berries, inc. millet, rice, etc.)

2 c boiling water

½ c ground grain

(Before use in home blender, grind grain fresh to the desired fineness or coarseness.)

ADD grain to pot of boiling water. STIR briskly to prevent lumping. Continue cooking over medium heat till thick. Lower heat and COOK slowly for 10 to 20 minutes.

Optional: add presoaked raisins, currants, etc.

ROLLED GRAINS (Barley, Oats, Rye, Wheat, etc)

2 cups boiling water

¾ c of the rolled grain

ADD grain to pot of boiling water. PLACE pot on medium heat and COOK slowly for 5 to 10 minutes. STIR only to keep heat uniform, NOT to change texture of the grain.

MILLET and CORNMEAL

5 c warm water

½ c millet

½ c coarse ground cornmeal

MIX and COOK in variety of ways:

    a. Crockpot overnight

    b. Casserole in oven for 1 hour at 350°

    c. Double boiler on stove top

    d. Heavy pot directly over burner, stirring frequently

EGYPTIAN FAVORITE

2 c boiling water

4 to 5 dates (cut in small pieces)

4 to 5 figs (cut in small pieces)

2 to 4 tbsp fresh ground cornmeal*

*Before adding, MOISTEN cornmeal with small amount of water to prevent lumps.

ADD dates and figs to water. COOK about 5 minutes. STIR in cornmeal to thicken. COOK slowly 10 to 20 minutes until grain is tender.

Crepes

REAL FOOD CREPE (a very thin pancake) — 30 Crepes (t)

Step 1 In electric blender ADD

2 c rolled baby oats	OR
½ c cornmeal	Use 3 c of any
½ c whole wheat flour	rolled grain
1 tsp salt	or flour

Step 2 ADD 3 to 3½ cups of very hot water to Step 1. WHIZ and blend well. Batter must be THIN! Each grain is different and a bit more water may be needed.

Step 3 BAKE as a therapeutic crepe. Go to **Step 5.**

Step 4 For a smoother crepe, let set overnight. Add from **1 to 4 whole eggs** and whiz again.

Step 5 BAKE: Heat a 6 to 8 inch heavy non-stick skillet till very hot! Pour a small amount of the crepe batter (2 tbsp) into skillet. Lift skillet from burner. Tilt from side to side and even upside-down to make sure no excess dough is in pan. Pour all excess back out. Return pan to heat. As soon as bubbles appear the crepe will be lightly brown on underside. Carefully lift edges all around crepe to be sure it is loose, then lift with a soft blade and turn. In about 10 seconds the other side will be done. Lift pan off burner and let crepe slide into storage oven, or on to a kitchen towel. Repeat for each crepe.

Step 6 ROLL or fold over **fruit,** or filling; top with sauce from page 6.

Step 7 May use with a **chicken** filling or use the sweet crepe recipe and make desserts. FREEZES WELL. Make in advance.

SWEET CREPE (*t*)... EXCELLENT!
Use **REAL FOOD CREPE recipe.**

Add **¼ to ½ c currants** or raisins to mixture and whiz again in blender till smooth and ground well; or soften the currants (as they are small) and leave them whole and stir into batter just before baking.

REMEMBER: Fruit like this will tend to make a crepe stick a bit, so practice and use a bit of no-stick if necessary.

WAFFLES (*t*)
Use **REAL FOOD CREPE recipe.**

Pour the batter into a HOT waffle iron which has been sprayed with a non-stick. Keep the batter thin! Leave batter in the iron from 10 to 12 minutes or until steaming stops. Must be completely cooked in order NOT to stick! Makes 6 medium sized round waffles.

REAL FOOD PANCAKES... Different and TASTY!
Step 1 Prepare **Steps 1, 2** and **4** of **Real Food Crepe.**

Step 2 ADD **one** whole peeled **ripe avocado.**
WHIZ until blended. Be sure batter is not too tight, as it must pour easily.

Step 3 BAKE as a pancake. Use 3 to 4 tbsp batter. Do not cover the whole bottom of baking pan as in "crepe", **Step 5.** TURN when fully baked and full of small holes on the upper side. Crepe will rise and be light and full.

REAL FOOD FRUIT PASTES — REAL FOOD JAMS (*t*)
Use for sweetenings, fillings, spreads

1. HEAT in saucepan **1 c dried fruits** (dates, currants, raisins, apple, fig, apricot, peach, pear, or other dried fruit.) with enough water to barely cover.
   Simmer slowly till all is soft mass.

   POUR all into food blender and whiz until smooth. Push down sides of blender as the mixture blends. Do not add all liquid at once. A bit at a time for blades to barely work. May not need all the liquid.

   Store in refrigerator . . . keep for all kinds of sweetening.

2. FRESH FRUIT JAM (fresh orchard picked in season)
   Place in blender and whir. Use at once.

3. OTHER JAMS:
   To No. 1 above, ADD **½ cup cranberries** cooked with the fruit or **1** cup unsweetened drained **pineapple.** (Use liquid in place of any water).

   For a tart jam, try mixing 1 whole well washed **orange,** rind and all, and/or ½ well washed **lemon.** CREATE!

4. CRANBERRY-ORANGE:
   12 to 16 oz fresh or **frozen cranberries,** cooked.
   WHIZ in blender with **1 whole washed orange.** Mix till well blended. For sweeter mix add ¼ **to** ½ **c fruit paste.**

FILLINGS FOR CREPES (tops for Waffles, Omelets, etc. (*t*)

1. Use **fresh fruit** from orchard or market. Mash in blender or process with blade into a sauce. Use fresh fruit as is.

2. Place a piece of whole **fresh fruit,** such as **banana,** inside crepe, roll and top with ample mashed fruit sauce.

3. Fruit, **canned in natural sauce,** or unsweetened frozen fruit:

continued next page

1 c fruit to **1 tbsp arrowroot** cooked only until thickened. Use as filling. For the topping use 1 c fruit to 2 tsp of arrowroot.

4. **1c** fresh or frozen **cranberries** (or other such fruit), **2 mejool dates** (or 1 tbsp fruit paste), ½ c water. Heat till berries crack or soften. Stir in blender till sauce. One **whole orange** including rind added to cranberry makes delicious marmalade.

5. Apple Syrup: **1 c reconstituted frozen applejuice.** Add **2 tsp arrowroot.** Mix and cook only till thickened and clear. OPTIONAL: Use maple flavoring, or other flavors of unsweetened frozen juices.

A Quickie

BREAKFAST MUFFINS (*t*)

METHOD ONE:

Step 1, 2, and 4 of Real Food Crepe recipe. May be thicker.

Step 5 ADD ¼ c **chopped dried fruit,** or currants, or raw cranberries; or create.

Step 6 POUR into teflon tiny muffin tin.

Step 7 Bake 350° for 20 to 30 minutes. Taste-test.

METHOD TWO:

Step 1 WHIZ **1 c finely shredded apple and 1 c finely rolled oats.**

Step 2 ADD **½ c currants,** or raisins, or date paste (and/or optional ½ c whizzed nuts).

Step 3 WHIZ all in food processor. ADD small amount of water if necessary (optional **1 or 2 eggs**).

Step 4 PACK into tiny teflon muffin tin.

Step 5 BAKE 375° for 25 minutes. Taste-test.

LUNCHEON IDEAS

SALADS

SOUPS

SANDWICH
- Use spreads and ideas from pages 78 on . . .
- Slice a vegetable, tomato, cuke, etc.
- Slice or mash an avocado . . . spread on toast
- Use sprouts generously
- Mash and season beans or lentils, spread on toast . . .

PIZZA
- Toast bread and top with cheese spread, p. 78 and real food sauce, p. 67, assorted sprouted grains, legumes, olives, seeds or nuts.

- Tear in half and make a sandwich

LIQUID SALADS or DRINKS

- No recipe given, create yourself

Salads

TABOULI — Salad or stuffing for pocket bread **(t)**

 1 c bulgar
¾ c fresh lemon juice
 2 bunches green scallions, tops and all (chopped)
 2 bunches chopped parsley tops
 2 large ripe peeled tomatoes (cut in pieces)
 1 large red or green sweet pepper (cubed in pieces)
 1 fresh cuke (cubed in small pieces)
 2 or 3 mashed garlic cloves
 1 tsp cumin seed (other herbs to taste)

SOFTEN BULGAR: Stir bulgar into 2 c briskly boiling water. Turn off heat, cover, and leave till all water is absorbed. May take 1 hour. OR (quick method), stir bulgar into 2 c briskly boiling water, then place over double boiler and keep warm for 20 minutes. STIR VERY GENTLY with fork to not soften texture of grain.

MIX: To swollen bulgar add the lemon juice. Then ADD all the other vegetables. CHILL. Keeps well.

BULGAR VARIATIONS (t) ... create yourself

Soften bulgar as shown above. Look in refrigerator and use whatever is in the inventory:

Onion ... chop into small pieces
Mint Leaves ... harvest a few from yard and chop fine
Cumin seed or powder ... for special taste
Spice or Herb ... whatever is desired
Finely chopped **tomato** in generous amounts
Finely chopped **celery, watercress, etc.**

Whatever vegetable is available can be finely chopped and added.

Be sure to add the fresh lemon juice to the warm bulgar first! Let stand a while and then add other spices and herbs and then the vegetables. Refrigerate—marinate. Keeps very well for many days.

Use other grains like Barley, Millet, etc.

SALAD VARIATIONS

1. **Sprouted lentils, sprouted mung beans, sprouted wheat,** etc. Serve mixed as a topping for finer sprouts such as **alfalfa.** Pour over a dressing of your choice.

2. Use **sprouted lentils,** etc., as a mixture for tossed salads along with **precooked beans** such as: black bean, great northern red bean, pink bean, lima bean, garbanzo, green, yellow, and snap beans.

3. **Rice** is excellent if cooked in advance and cooled. Can be added to any processed or tossed salad for a hearty meal. (Same for **any legume** or **any bean.**)

4. Blend: peeled **broccoli stems, cauliflower, celery root, lemon slice,** with blade in the food processor. Add to any salad.

5. Sprinkle salad with **sesame seed, sunflower seed, blossoms** from spring vegetables such as mustard, etc.

6. Get acquainted with **wild weeds** which are edible in the early spring when tender. Use them. Contact local college teachers or the Farm Extension Offices.

7. Look for new vegetables in the market. Vary the diet . . . use something new!

8. Fix an old favorite . . . in a NEW way!

JOANNE'S IDEA (*t*)

Mix together:　Some **cold cooked rice**
　　　　　　　chopped **parsley** or watercress
　　　　　　　small pieces cut **celery**
　　　　　　　small cubes **cucumber**
　　　　　　　bean sprouts

Create your own proportions. **Soy sauce** enhances the flavor. Mix dressing of your choice from pages 77-80.

REAL FOOD SAUTÉ SALAD (*t*)
A main dish serving 2 people

½ chopped red sweet onion (green or other)
1 c mushrooms cut in half
1 head leaf lettuce cut in strips or coarsely chopped
1 large tomato cut and cubed
  other garden greens as desired
2 cups cooked rice
  sprouts
  lemon thyme

Sauté mushrooms quickly in dry, ungreased teflon pan, just barely browning. Remove from heat and add onions; let marinate. Sauté damp lettuce in very hot pan briefly, stirring constantly (only wilt). Add the mushrooms and onions. Remove from heat and cover. Warm the rice in microwave.

ARRANGE: Set out the salad plates. Place large pinch of sprouts on one corner, the sautéed greens on another corner, and the rice on another corner. Sprinkle cut tomato over everything, and add other greens such as **parsley, watercress, celantro, green pepper,** etc. Add seeds of choice. Cover rice with a generous sprinkle of **lemon thyme.** Sprinkle **garlic powder over all.** Serve with **toasted Real Food Bread** for a complete meal.

OPTIONAL: Cold cubed **fowl** or **fish** may be added to the corner of the salad beside the rice. Sprinkle fish with **lemon juice.**

MOCK GELATIN SALAD (*t*)

1 large carrot, cubed
½ banana (fresh or frozen)
½ sweet green pepper*

Use food processor and finely grate with a blade till a nice congealed mass. Serve on lettuce leaf or in compote glass. *May use other such as: apple, avocado, or fruit to taste.

12

Green Garden Salads

(using a food processor)

1. GRATED CARROT — 2 generous servings

t Shred (or grate with blade) **1 whole large carrot.** Shred with medium disc **1 peeled quartered apple.** Thinly slice a **stalk of celery** using slicing blade. Run a piece of **lemon** through processor. Mixture in the bowl will be a combination of fruits, vegetables and juices. Very little seasoning will be needed. For texture some **crushed fresh pineapple** can be added. A few **currants** or **presoaked raisins** can be added. (For a fruit dressing, combine low-fat yogurt with ½ of mashed banana in blender.)

2. GARDEN VEGETABLE — 2 generous servings

t (Vary with what is available on market or in garden.) Use blade in processor bowl and add the following cut vegetables: 1 small **cubed onion,** 1 whole mashed **garlic,** 1 full slice **lemon,** ½ sweet **green pepper,** 1 medium **cuke,** 1 tender **celery stalk,** fresh **herbs** from garden, 3 or 4 **snap peas,** cut up green leaves from **watercress,** garden **mustard,** or **spinach,** and ½ of a fresh peeled **tomato.** Blend till all are barely chopped. Remove blade. Add another ½ tomato cut in small pieces. Serve on bed of sprouts or in a peeled tomato shell. Make dressing using food blender. Blend a small amount of each of the salad ingredients including tomato until in a liquid form. Add **lemon.** Pour over as a dressing.

3. TOSSED SALAD

t Take any regular tossed salad mixture, containing large hunks of **iceberg lettuce,** drop into food processor with blade, ½ c or so at a time. Blend very slightly with blade. Remove and repeat, until all of salad hunks are processed into small pieces. If **lemon juice** and pieces of lemon are left in tossed salad at beginning of blending a delightful taste will result. Serve at once on shredded or broken tender pieces of lettuce. Top with vegetables or parsley.

REAL FOOD POTATO SALAD

Step 1 Cook till tender **5 medium potatoes** in skins.

Step 2 Prepare in large mixing bowl:

    1 c finely diced celery
    1 small can sliced olives
    2 oz diced pimiento
    1 tbsp onion powder or 2 tbsp onion flakes
    ¼ c chopped parsley
    ¼ c chopped red or green sweet pepper
    ½ c chopped green onions and tops
    Herbs to taste
  ½ tsp paprika
    1 tsp fresh lemon thyme
    1 tbsp dill seed
    1 tsp cumin seed
    1 tsp to 1 tbsp lemon juice
    Salt to taste (1 tsp)
  ½ to ¾ c low-fat yogurt (1 g per c, or
    REAL FOOD Yogurt)

Step 3 Peel or leave skins on potato. Dump drained cooked potatoes on top of Step 2 (chopped vegetables, etc.). With a sharp knife cut the potato into small pieces. Then take a flat mixing whip and continue to cut the potato into the vegetables. A sharp knife will do but takes a bit longer. Then stir till potato is all mixed and partly mashed into the vegetable mixture. CHILL or serve warm.

NOTE: For Therapeutic level, omit yogurt and add more **lemon juice.**

BEAN SALAD (*t*)

Follow any conventional mixed bean salad for ingredients. Omit all oil and vinegar. Use **Real Food Base** (p. 77-80) with herbs to taste for the dressing. Create!

GREEN VEGETABLE SALAD — not always lettuce! (*t*)

1 full slice cubed or ½ of a sweet pepper
3 inches of a cuke, cubed
1 stalk green onion (or 1 slice of red sweet onion)
1 small mashed garlic clove
1 tender stalk and top of celery, cubed
4 stalks watercress, celantro, spinach, or substitute
1 peeled ripe tomato, cubed

COMBINE all above in bowl, and squeeze with hands before adding the tomato. Add **herbs** to taste. Add dressing, or sprinkle **lemon juice** over all. Serve on plate of **sprouts.** 2 generous servings.

Soups

BARLEY-VEGETABLE SOUP (*t*)

8 c water (or broth of leftovers)
⅓ c whole grain barley
COOK for 1 hour or until tender.

ADD:
1 c sliced carrot
½ c tops and sliced stalks celery
½ c chopped or sliced onion
3 whole tomatoes broken in small pieces
COOK until just tender ... remove from stove and
ADD:
1 c frozen peas

SERVE and garnish with bits of **parsley, watercress,** etc.

VERY QUICK SOUPS (t)

Step 1 Inventory refrigerator or freezer. **Frozen peas,** fresh asparagus, broccoli, mushrooms, corn, etc.

Step 2 For Pea Soup (as an example): Cook peas till barely done.

Step 3 Transfer to food blender or processor with blade and whiz till well blended.

Step 4 Add seasonings: Dry chopped **onion, garlic,** mixed dry **herbs** to taste, chopped **parsley.**

Step 5 If a thickened soup is desired add arrowroot or whole wheat flour mixed into water (see p. 74).

Step 6 Reheat and SERVE.

NOTE: Any fresh or frozen vegetable can be made into a "quickie" soup with above method.

WHITE BEAN SOUP (t)

Wash well and soak **1 lb white (great northern) beans** overnight.

Next morning:

Cook in 8 c water about 1½ hours to soften.
Saute **2 c onion** in ¼ c water.

ADD: **2 c cut carrots**
1 c cut celery and tops
2 fresh sieved tomatoes

When beans are soft, or skin breaks add the vegetables and seasoning to taste. Simmer with beans and vegetables about 15 to 20 minutes until vegetables become tender. Garnish with sprigs of **parsley.**

TURKEY/CHICKEN or GIBLET BROTH

Put **meat pieces** or **giblets** in kettle and cover with water. Cook slowly several hours or all day. Cool. Remove bones from meat and discard all unwanted bones and/or meats. CHILL in refrigerator until firm. Lift and remove all fat which has risen to top and discard. Use gelatin like broth as base for soups, entrées, etc.

POTATO SOUP (*t*)

    1 c peeled, cubed potato
    1 c chopped onion
    1 c chopped celery and leaves

Sauté onion in small amount of water, add rest of vegetables and 4 c water (or broth). Add spice and **herbs** to taste. When tender mash the vegetables to make them soft. Simmer. Sprinkle with **parsley** to garnish when serving.

REAL FOOD MINESTRONE (*t*)

Prepare:
    1 c cooked lima beans
    1 c cooked kidney beans
    ½ c cooked whole barley

Sauté **1 whole chopped onion** in ¼ c water in kettle.

ADD:
    1½ cups diced celery
    ½ c diced parsley
    3 quarts whole tomatoes and juice (generous)
    1 bay leaf
    1 clove garlic
    2 c (chopped and mixed carrot, zucchini, potato, green beans, green pepper, corn or other vegetables on hand

Cook until tender and ADD

    1 c cooked lima beans
    1 c cooked kidney beans
    ½ c cooked whole barley
    ½ c raw whole wheat elbow or short macaroni
    salt and herbs to taste.

Cook till tender. SERVE with sprinkle of parsley.

GREEK LENTIL (*t*)

1 onion chopped and sautéed in ¼ c water in large saucepan.
ADD:
- **1 medium chopped carrot**
- **1 chopped celery stalk**
- **1 small cubed potato**
- **2 c uncooked lentils**
- **8 c water** or broth)
- **2 bay leaves**

Bring to simmering boil and cook only until tender, about one hour.

Just before serving, ADD:
- **1 tsp salt**
- **2 tsp fresh lemon juice**

REAL FOOD MIXED BEAN SOUP - STEW (*t*)

Soak overnight: **½ c each:**
- **Ming Bean**
- **Navy Bean**
- **Red Kidney Bean**
- **Pink Bean**
- **Great Northern**
- **Other**

Next morning: Rinse well. Place in large pot and cover the beans with at least 1 inch of water. Cook about 1½ to 2 hours until tender. Taste test.

Sauté **1 cup chopped onion** in ¼ c water.

ADD: **2 to 4 c chopped vegetables** from refrigerator **(celery, carrot, turnip, peppers, greens, etc.)**.

ADD: **2 to 4 cups of whole stewed tomatoes.**
Continue cooking till all vegetables are tender. Use herbs and salt to taste. SERVE.

18

CORN CHOWDER

SOAK overnight: ¼ c dry navy beans, 4 c water.

Or use alternative: Simmer very slowly for 1 hour.

DRAIN, RINSE; then cover navy beans with water and cook for 1 to 2 hours or till very soft.

WHIZ in food blender until smooth. Set aside.

SAUTE 1 c chopped onions in ¼ c water.

ADD 1 c diced potatoes, and 1 c water. Cook until tender. Then whiz in blender until smooth.

ADD to blender: 1½ c fresh corn kernels (or freshly defrosted kernels). Whiz until smooth.

ADD the smooth beans.

ADD: 1 c raw skim milk and 1 tsp salt.

RETURN to heat and

ADD ¼ c whole corn kernels.

Heat to slow simmer for about 20 minutes. SERVE.

(For a richer chowder use ¼ raw cream)

SOUP DUMPLINGS (or Stew Dumplings)

1 c whole wheat flour
1 whole egg
dash of salt if desired
¼ c water or soup stock

MIX all together with whip until blended.

ADD any additional water to make a thick smooth batter. Drop by small teaspoons into soup, while it is slowly boiling. Continue to simmer for 10 to 20 minutes until dumpling is cooked through. Taste test!

BREADS

CRACKERS

MISCELLANEOUS

REAL FOOD GROUND GRAIN BREAD, fat and sugar-free, makes 4 to 5 1-lb. loaves (*t*)

Step 1   MILL or purchase and warm **10 to 12 c** of a **hard winter wheat.**

Step 2   MIX together and set aside to rise (in a 2 c measure)
¾ cup warm water (110°)
½ tsp applejuice concentrate or
        diastatic malt (p. 34)
     2 tbsp active yeast

Step 3   In blender WHIZ **1 large ripe apple** in 1 c hot water. (Or, substitute apple with either ½ c pitted dates or ½ to ¾ c frozen unsweetened apple concentrate) ADD enough very **warm water** to make 5 cups.

Step 4   **(If by hand skip to Step 8).**
POUR the Blender Mix (Step 3) into bowl, start mixing, ADD 5 to 8 c of warm flour slowly for even mixing without lumps. MIX with mixer for a full 5 minutes to start the gluten in the flour, working in the dough.

ADD the Yeast Mixture (Step 2) which has bubbled up to more than twice its size. (If it has not made bubbles, it is no good. Repeat Step 2.) Stir yeast mixture before adding. Continue with the electric mixer and ADD 2-3 more cups of warm flour. ADD **1 to 2 tbsp salt** to taste. MIX 5 full minutes.

ADD just enough additional flour, 1-2 cups, so dough cleans sides of mixing bowl. Each milling of flour is different, so amounts need to be adjusted. When the dough holds together in a ball and the sides of bowl stir clean, enough flour has been added. DO NOT ADD EXTRA; DOUGH NEEDS TO BE SOFT. MIX about 5 more minutes. Drop out onto a floured board for shaping into loaves.

Step 5 SHAPING: Prepare pans with a non-stick, then sprinkle with cornmeal over sides and bottom. May weigh each loaf to fit pan: i.e., 1¼ lbs. for 7 x 3 x 2½ pan; 1¾ lbs for a 10 x 3 x 2½ pan. Fill baking pan ⅓ to ½ with dough. Cut dough into equal parts to fit pans available. Flatten each section slightly and roll into shape of pan (if new to breadmaking, see footnote). After loaves are weighed and shaped into pans, the center of the loaf can be cut with a sharp knife full length of the loaf and **sesame seeds** sprinkled over the top, or as the loaves are shaped and prepared, they can be rolled in sesame seed for a covering, then placed in the pan. If a braided loaf is desired; flatten one loaf slightly and cut into three ropes, but leave joined at one end; then braid, leaving cut side up to show and pinch at the end, sealing all three ropes together. Tuck ends under and lay in pan. See Step 7.

Step 6 Reserve Dough for refrigerator.
Put extra dough into a plastic bag and refrigerate for: crackers, p. 33; pocket bread, p. 26; breakfast rolls, p. 28, etc.

Step 7 RAISING before baking: Place the filled pans with the dough to be raised in your oven (or other draft-free place). DO NOT TURN ON OVEN HEAT YET. Allow at least ½ hour for the dough to double in bulk and reach tops of the pans. Allow more time if needed. With bread already in oven as it rises, turn on oven to 350° and BAKE for 35-45 minutes or until the bread falls free of pan when inverted and has a nice crust. Cover for 1 hour with a clean cloth. When cool, store in airtight bag in cool place until ready to eat. Freezing destroys E vitamins. Shelf life un-refrigerated 3 to 5 days depending upon the weather. Whole wheat bread dries quickly when a cut loaf is exposed to the air!

Step 8 MIXING BY HAND **(Optional):**
Use above measurements. Pour blender mix into bowl, add flour to start gluten working. Add yeast mixture. Add enough flour so as to work bread with hands in a kneading process. (For detailed instructions, ask your County Home Extension Agent for copy of sheet, called: "Breadmaking.")* Knead till the dough becomes elastic and then cover the dough and let rest and it doubles in size and bulk. Work again, and knead WELL. Shape into loaves by dividing into 4 or 6 loaves, depending upon size of pans. Shape loaves to fit pan. Follow above raising-baking directions.

Step 9 BREAD—Variations
Milling: Several different kinds of grains can be milled to make a multi-grain loaf of bread. Millet, cornmeal, oats, oatmeal, barley, rolled barley, rye, etc., or even a 9 grain cereal can be used. Use grains ground, rolled, or even sprouted. Cornmeal is a good grain to clean the bowl in a final mixing. Corn is used in the mill to clean the stones. ADDITIONAL GRAINS MAKE FOR A HEAVIER BREAD AND ADJUSTMENTS OFTEN NEED TO BE MADE. Use variations a little at a time, until you understand what you are doing!

BLENDING: Fruits, or vegetables blended and used as liquid, are fine. Sprouted grains, lentils, soya, etc., crushed with blades in food processor or heavy duty blender first. Use ¾ to ½ c of raisins and blend with apple. Use sunflower or sesame seed. Whole millet, and amaranth stirred into batter is great.

*Or, write your yeast company, or visit local library, illustrated breadmaking books are available. Adapt this FAT-, SUGAR-FREE method to existing illustrated breadmaking recipes.

REAL FOOD SPROUTED GRAINS BREAD (t) . . . a generous loaf; very tasty, but not good form; toasts well.

Step 1 Assemble:

   2 c wheat berries (sprouted for 48 hours).
   1 tbsp yeast
   ½ tsp diastatic malt
   ¼ tsp salt to taste
   1 to 2 c fresh ground warm whole wheat flour

Step 2 Place sprouted berries in home food blender (or use the blade in heavy duty food processor). ADD a drop or two of hot water for blades to operate, if necessary.

BLEND on HEAVY speed, pushing down often with scraper, until the whole mass is well blended into a batter, (or put through a meat grinder).

Step 3 ADD yeast and malt. Blend. ADD salt. Blend.

Step 4 At this step the dough can be baked in pan on top of stove, pancake style, or in oven, cake style.

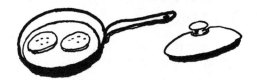

Step 5 STIR in additional flour to make a soft ball until the dough seems to leave sides of bowl.

Step 6 COVER and let RISE for about ½ hour or so.

Step 7 STIR briskly. ADD a bit of flour if necessary. Do not make too stiff a batter. Keep light and soft. Let RISE again for ½ hour or doubled.

Step 8 STIR and SHAPE into loaf. Roll loaf in **sesame seeds.**

Step 9 Follow general directions for BREAD and BAKING on pages 22, 23, 24.

NO FAIL . . . REAL FOOD POCKET BREAD (*t*)

Step 1 RESERVE dough from REAL FOOD basic bread.

Step 2 CUT and DIVIDE dough into equal portions, using about ½ cup each. Set aside, cover to keep moisture in the dough.

Step 3 Secure EQUIPMENT.*

Step 4 SEE ILLUSTRATION. Place a ball of dough in the center of four lids on a breadboard. Using a rolling pin, ROLL evenly to form a circle of the dough. ROLL to ⅛ of an inch thick and about 5 to 8 inches across. When the rolling pin and the lids meet, the dough is the right thickness!

Step 5 Place each flat loaf as it is rolled onto a wooden surface or on a cloth-covered flat surface. When the cloth is filled with loaves, each laying without touching another, cover with a clean cloth to keep dampness in the loaves. **If dry weather, mist the air** with a bit of water over the top cloth. Loaves must remain a bit moist, but not wet!

Step 6 BAKING: Prepare the oven with four 6" or 8" squares of UNGLAZED QUARRY TILE on the bottom shelf. Heat oven and tiles to 450° or 500°.

Step 7 When oven is prepared and HOT, carefully lift each loaf with the palm of hand and turn into oven directly on the hot tile without disturbing the loaf and dough unnecessarily. Close oven at once. Dough will begin to RISE and loaf will "pocket." **Do not leave in oven more than 3 minutes!** Remove and place another loaf in the hot oven to bake.

*EQUIPMENT FOR MAKING POCKET BREAD

4 to 6 mason-type sealing jar lids
a rolling pin
a spray mister with water
several large dish drying towels
a large flat space to store the loaves before baking
unglazed quarry tile for the oven
a large thin metal spatula if possible (to lift loaves)

OTHER IDEAS:

The little loaf "pocket" does not need to be turned while it is baking.

Pocket can be eaten at once, as soon as it cools to the touch . . . or stored as Real Food Bread is stored. For a sandwich, tear apart as in illustration and make into two equal pieces, for two sandwiches.

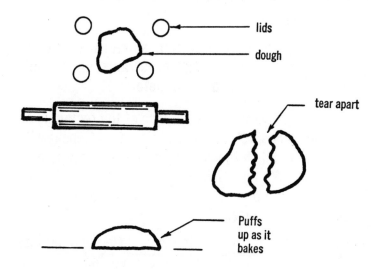

lids

dough

tear apart

Puffs up as it bakes

REAL FOOD BREAD DOUGH . . . HINTS

Store the fresh dough in refrigerator, in a clean plastic bag for up to 1 week. Remove and bring to room temperature before being formed into pastry. Place in a microwave oven on defrost till dough is warm and comes to life.

REAL FOOD BREAKFAST ROLLS (*t* if nuts omitted)

One pound of Real Food Bread Dough, p. 22, will make two generous Danish-type pastry rolls. (For a sweeter dough add more sweetening when making basic dough on p. 22)

Step 1 ROLL ½ lb of the dough onto a flat floured surface, rectangle shape, about ½ inch thick. Roll to about 8 x 10 or 10 x 12 inches. Keep light flour on board under the dough just to prevent sticking as it is rolled. Keep the dough light! Do not work in extra amounts of flour. (May roll dough directly into baking pan, thus no need to lift the finished roll into pan after it is finished.)

Step 2 **Prepare a jam mixture as shown on p. 6** to use for the filling.

Step 3 When the dough is rolled flat, spread with Step 2. Sprinkle with **softened raisins, currants,** and/or **nutmeats** as desired. Season to taste.

Step 4 ROLL. (a) Starting at each side of the rectangle on the long sides, roll to center, like a rug. Repeat with other side. Pinch the ends up to form a boat to hold the fruits. With a brush or spatula, spread additional jam or paste or juices over exposed dough on the outside for a glaze.

(b) OPTION . . . Roll all the way closed and cut into 1″ slices, like a snail. Lay in prepared (as for bread, p. 23) cookie sheets or teflon pan.

(c) OPTION . . . Roll and shape as desired. Create.

Step 5 RAISE. Let stand till double in size and light, about 30 minutes in warm location. If it appears to be drying out, spray with very fine mist of water, very lightly.

Step 6 BAKE: 350° oven directly on a quarry tile base if preferred, for 20 to 30 minutes. Or in oven on rack. Watch and test!

Step 7 EAT: Eat while still warm and fresh. Whole wheat, freshly ground, dries out quickly when baked and exposed to fresh air. Cover and wrap when cool. Leave at room temperature for 2 to 3 days.

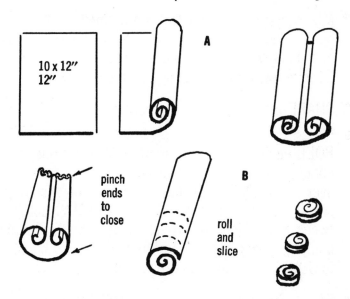

RICE CRACKER

ROLL **2 cups freshly cooked brown rice** between 2 pieces of handiwrap. Spread on a bit of cornmeal to prevent sticking.

TRANSFER to teflon (non-stick) baking sheet.

BAKE for 45 minutes at 300° until crisp or brown. Taste test. Score into 2 x 2 squares.

ALTERNATIVE:

1. ADD 4 tbsp ground **sesame seed** to above before rolling.
2. ADD 1 tbsp **onion flakes** before rolling.
3. ADD **herb** seasoning to taste.
4. CREATE YOUR OWN MIXTURE!

REAL FOOD WHOLE WHEAT FLOUR TORTILLA (*t*)

Step 1 DOUGH:

    1 c freshly ground wheat berries (flour)

    ¼ c freshly ground sesame seeds (or nuts)

      (use home blender machine)

    sprinkle of salt as desired

    ½ to ⅓ c hot water

Step 2 MIX enough hot water to form a soft ball. Work in palm of hand for a few minutes. WRAP in plastic bag or in handiwrap. Let stand and rest for 10 minutes. Open and work in hands again, like a ball.

Step 3 SHAPE into four equal pieces. Cover to keep from drying out.

ROLL each piece into a small 8-9 inch circle, and about 1/16 of an inch thick; lift the dough and turn over each roll. Dough should not stick on a smooth wooden surface. USE FLOUR SPARINGLY. Roll between two pieces of waxed paper similar to pie dough.) When each piece has been rolled, be sure to COVER with towel to prevent drying!

Step 4 BAKE: Prepare a very HOT heavy skillet and use no fat. Keep pan dry. Lay one tortilla in the hot pan and wait for small bubbles to appear. Tortilla will brown in spots on underside. Turn and repeat on opposite side. Cooks quickly. Taste test. (A heavy cast iron or aluminum is best.) Wrap each piece in a cotton cloth as it is baked, carefully folding cloth over to keep covered. Serve warm or with salads, or make Burrito, as follows. A good, fast hot bread for lots of meals, or picnics.

REAL FOOD BURRITO (*t* level depending on filling)

Step 1 Prepare Tortillas.

Step 2 Lay the fresh, soft tortilla on a working surface, spread **2 to 3 tbsp of mashed seasoned beans** through the center portion. Fold over one side to cover the beans. See illustration. Then fold each end to form an oblong sandwich. Practice the fold until each side is folded independently to form a tight sandwich. See illustration.

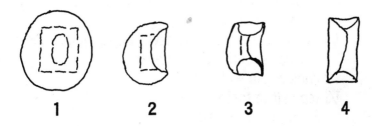

1　　　　**2**　　　　**3**　　　　**4**

Step 3 Wrap in wax paper, foil, or place in a covered dish. Reheat in moderate oven, or microwave on reheat. Serve.

Step 4 ALTERNATE fillings may be made instead of using beans. Season with **chopped green chili, salsa sauce,** etc. Create!

REAL FOOD BREAD STICKS (*t*)

Use some of the reserved **Real Food Ground Grain Bread Dough.** Measure ¼ c or less dough for each stick. Divide dough and set aside. Roll each piece of ¼ c dough into shape of a fat pencil about 6 to 8 inches long. Place each piece into teflon pan. Let rise. Bake slowly, 300° oven, till crisp and/or complete the baking after turning oven off till sticks are dried in the oven. Stores well on shelf. May be rolled in **sesame, poppy, celery, or any tasty seed or herb** before baking.

REAL FOOD WHOLE WHEAT BATTER BREAD, (*t*) real easy, no kneading. Developed for my bachelor son.

Step 1 MIX and let work in a draft-free warm area:
   ⅔ c warm water, 110°
   2 tbsp active fresh dry yeast
   1 tsp frozen unsweetened apple concentrate
   Put into a 2 c measure.

Step 2 MILL **5 c whole wheat berries** or warm **whole wheat flour** in oven.

Step 3 In large heavy bowl to hold warmth, MIX:
   5 c warmed flour
   ½ to ¾ c concentrated unsweetened apple juice
   (or use substitute sweetener)
   2 cups warm water, 110°
   ¼ tsp salt to taste
   STIR and MIX well.

Step 4 ADD the yeast which has now bubbled up and just about filled the 2 c measure.

Step 5 BEAT and MIX well and add any **additional flour** to make a batter which will pour but still seems to have life and body, sort of slippery-heavy type batter. (May add wheat germ, cornmeal, millet, amaranth, oatmeal, etc.) Use common sense and train the eye.

Step 6 Prepare baking pan as for bread, p. 23. Pour or spoon batter into pan. Fill ½ full. Use 2 lb pan, or two 1-lb pans.

Step 7 Let the dough now rise in draft-free place till it is doubled or reaches top of pan. (Place in unheated oven.)

Step 8 Turn heat to 375°. BAKE for from 35 to 45 minutes until bread will fall free from pan. Follow directions on page 23.

CORNMEAL CRACKERS

Step 1 1 c fresh fine ground corn
2 tbsp sesame seed
1 cup BOILING water

Step 2 Prepare pan for crackers. Use teflon cookie sheet, or spray non-stick on regular pan.

Step 3 PLACE 1 c cornmeal in bowl. ADD 2 tbsp sesame seed. Have a whipping wand ready and quickly pour in the BOILING water; WHIP and mix well, keeping the batter warm.

Step 4 Quickly drop the dough onto the sheet, and with wet palms press the dough throughout the sheet in a flat, smooth manner. Dough will be hot; keep it that way. When level, sprinkle with salt, or herbs to taste, and push in with palms. With the back of a spatula or rubber scraper, cut diagonal lines through the pan to separate into small 2-inch diamond squares before baking.

Step 5 Bake 350° until golden brown. Watch, as each batch differs according to the corn used, moisture absorbed, and thickness of each.

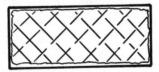

REAL FOOD CRACKERS (*t*)

Follow above directions, using **other ground grains and seasonings of choice.**

OR . . . roll out **Real Food Bread Dough 1/16 to ¼ inch thick** and lay in teflon pan. Score into shape, sprinkle on seasonings. Mist spray with water before baking at 325 to 350° for 10 to 15 minutes.

REAL FOOD FAST BREAD STIX (*t*)

Cut a **slice of Real Food Bread** or cut slice of market purchased non-fat Ezekiel-type bread into strips the size of one finger. Arrange in baking pan and **sprinkle with seasonings of onion powder, garlic powder, herbs, etc.** Spray with water to hold . . . toast in oven till crisp.

REAL FOOD CROUTONS (*t*)

Cut **bread** into small cubes . . . mist or spray with water . . . sprinkle on **herbs** and **spice** . . . bake till crisp. Stores well.

DIASTATIC MALT (*t*)

Soak **1 c of wheat berries (or barley) overnight.** Drain and let sprout, cleaning with fresh water two or three times each day. When sprouts are showing about ½ inch, drain and dry in a warm oven, 110 to 120°. When VERY dry, run them through a clean mill. The result will be a very fine flour that tastes like malt. A heavy duty blender may do a less successful, but adequate job. Cover tightly, and store in refrigerator. Use in breads for sweetening. Use as sweetening in other recipes and to roll REAL FOOD "candy" in.

DEXTRINIZING

The changing of carbohydrates to dextrins.
Heat dry in oven or in skillet, **Rice, Barley, Wheat,** etc.

Stir in skillet for from 3 to 5 minutes. Some grains pop when cooked. In the oven, allow to bake at 325° for 5 to 10 minutes. Watch to see it does not burn. Most grains will turn a delicate brown. Dextrinizing shortens the cooking time of grains, as well as making them sweeter.

Prepare in advance and store in refrigerator or pantry shelf.

SWEETS
CRUSTS FOR PIES AND COMPOTES

FILLINGS FOR PIE

A BASIC DOUGH

CAKES

MISCELLANEOUS

Crusts for Pies and Compotes

For all **baked** crusts in this book — pie will need to **Tenderize** for several hours by being covered tightly. Place in a tupperware type sealer, or, turn a large bowl upside down over pie, cool and place in refrigerator 24 to 48 hours to tenderize crust.

APPLE AND OAT CRUST (*t*)

Step 1   Grate or shred **1½ c apple.**
Grind **1 c rolled oats** in blender till fine.

Step 2   Mix oat flour and grated apple together till ball forms. Can use food processor.

Step 3   Use teflon pan, or spray non-stick.

Step 4   Drop ball of dough into pan. Cover hand with plastic bag and press into shape of pan. If a lid is desired, save some dough to flatten and spread over top.

Step 5   Flatten dough between two pieces of plastic wrap, or bags, or with hands, and strip over top of pie.

Step 6   BAKE:
(a) For shell only . . . 350°, 20-25 minutes. Fill with hot filling and tenderize for 12-24 hours.

(b) Shell for 10 to 15 minutes, fill with cooked filling, carefully spread reserved dough over top, lattice fashion. Return to oven and bake till covering is done.

MULTIPURPOSE PIE SHELL
SEE page 45 for "pie."

BREAD AND FRUIT PIE CRUST (t) . . . a favorite standby REAL FAST, AND REAL GOOD!

Step 1 Prepare bread crumbs. Fresh soft ones. WHIZ **3 to 4 slices REAL FOOD Bread** in blender or food processor.

Step 2 Soften **4 to 6 pitted Mejool dates.** Or use about ½ **cup date or fruit paste** (see page 74), (banana or other sweet fruit, or frozen juice concentrate. Adjust amounts for sweetness desired.)

Step 3 Blend the sweetening into the bread crumbs to form a softened mass which will press into pie pan.

Step 4 Drop into pie pan. Cover hand with plastic bag and shape crust. Will flute if pressed into shape.

Step 5 Fill at once with choice of fillings. Or . . .
(a) Bake, fill, then tenderize.
(b) Press into individual compote serving dishes, fill with choice of fillings.
(c) Layer with fruit in individual serving dishes.
(d) See Strawberry Shortcake, p. 49.

OPTIONALS:
Add 2 tbsp crushed almonds, or 2 tbsp coconut or ¼ c rolled barley or rolled oats to Step 1 for different texture. Create!

ALMOND PIE CRUST

Step 1 **1 to 2 c ground roasted almonds**
3 to 6 tbsp rolled barley (add with almonds)
2 to 4 tbsp water (or liquid)

Step 2 WHIZ nuts and barley in blender or food processor. Add non-irritating spice to taste. Whiz in enough liquid to form a nice ball of crust.

Step 3 PRESS crust into pie shell evenly. BAKE at 350° for 30 to 40 minutes. Do not overbake or burn! Will make one extra large, tender pie crust or two smaller ones.

NUT AND BARLEY DELICIOUSLY TENDER CRUST
(Rolled Crust)

Step 1 1 c barley flour (whiz flakes or mill whole grains)
½ tsp salt
1 c roasted cashews (brazil, or other nut), blended
until smooth
½ c water or liquid

Step 2 Prepare above and mix. ADD the water until a nice ball is formed. Use processor or mix by hand.

Step 3 ROLL pastry crust in traditional manner. Use two pieces of waxed paper and a bit of barley flour to prevent sticking. Keep turning paper and dough to roll evenly. Lift paper carefully, adding additional barley flour to keep dough from sticking. Dough will be very tender and fragile, BUT it mends easily! Make crust and top. Use paper to lift crust into pan, and to place crust on top if desired.

Step 4 BAKE pie and let tenderize for up to 24 hours before eating to be sure liquid of pie completely penetrates the crust.

COCONUT PIE SHELL

Step 1 WHIZ till smooth 1 c shredded coconut, 1 tbsp barley, rice or wheat flour.

Step 2 ADD enough liquid only to make a ball of dough.

Step 3 Put plastic bag over hand and press dough into teflon pie pan, or use non-stick on pan.

Step 4 BAKE 350° for 10 to 15 minutes. Or bake in glass pan in microwave oven.

FRUIT PIE SHELL FOR FROZEN DELIGHTS in a crust (*t* if nuts omitted)

Step 1 WHIZ and mix:
  1 c date paste
  ⅓ c finely grated coconut
  1 tbsp cranberry/orange relish, p. 6
  ½ c finely chopped nutmeats

Step 2 Spread fruit paste all around the pie shell evenly. Sprinkle nuts over the crust and press in evenly. FREEZE. Shell should be thin and even throughout the pan.

Step 3 Fill crust with fruits or a cream pie filling (strawberries or kiwi). Freeze.

IDEAS: Try new ideas. Crush some **puffed rice.** Line pie shell with **moist fruit** and press puffed rice into the fruit. Do not bake.

Fillings for Pie

Choose a crust; then choose a filling . . .

APPLE and RAISIN

Step 1 Peel, core and finely slice **4 to 6 large pie apples.**

Step 2 MIX Step 1 in large cooking pot with:
  ¼ to ½ cup raisins or currants
  ½ c mashed dates, or 8 large Mejool dates
  1 tsp ground coriander
  ½ tsp ground anise
  2 to 3 tsp arrowroot* with ½ to¾ cup water **or frozen apple concentrate** to thicken the liquid that results from cooking. (More may need to be added!)

Step 3 continued next page

Step 3 COOK until clear and pour into pie shell. Serve. **Top with glaze,** or a cream. (See chapter on glazes and creams.)

OPTION: Cook till apples are tender and almost done. Pour into a Pie Crust, cover with a top crust and bake till crust is done.

For a single crust baked Apple Pie, top with an Apple or an **Orange Glaze.**

***Tapioca:** Use finely ground Tapioca in place of arrowroot, and cook till tapioca becomes clear and tender. Adds a nice texture to the filling.

NOTE: **Measurements need not be exact** for the fruit pastes, or the grains in most of the recipes in this book. Generalities will often bring excellent results ... hence the often vague measurements in some of the recipes. Use different amounts and CREATE!

My grandmother always said every recipe needed several ounces of comon sense. Good advice!

BANANA CREAM PIE

WITHOUT NUTS (*t*)	WITH NUTS
2 c water	½ c roasted cashews
1 t vanilla	2 c water
1 c date paste	1 t vanilla
4 to 4½ tbsp arrowroot	1 c date paste
	4 to 4½ tbsp arrowroot
	salt to taste

Step 1 WHIZ all ingredients in the food blender until very smooth.

Step 2 Cook over low heat until mixture thickens, stirring to keep batter smooth. COOL.

Step 3 Select **3 large bananas** and PREPARE **coconut crust,** p. 38 (or crust of choice).

Step 4 Slice banana. Spread over bottom of crust, then spread with filling. Repeat until full. (Or, stir sliced bananas into cooled filling and pour into crust. Sprinkle top with **finely grated coconut.** CHILL for up to 12 or 24 hours.

OPTIONAL: Stir **4 oz. of Real Food Cheese** into filling before pouring in crust.

CHERRY PIE

Step 1 **1 quart pitted cherries.** Drain and reserve the liquid.

Step 2 To each cup of liquid add **2 tbsp arrowroot** powder. Add spice to taste. Pour into pot and slowly bring to heat.

Step 3 Cook until clear, stirring to keep smooth. When thickened, remove from heat and cool.

Step 4 ADD ½ c **Kefir cheese,** REAL FOOD cheese or Neufchatel cheese. WHIZ until smooth.

Step 5 Stir drained cherries into Step 4, and then pour into pie shell. Tenderize for 24 hours.

Step 6 Top with **glaze** of choice.

> Note: For a strawberry pie: cook a few strawberries to make the 1 cup liquid in which to add 2 TB arrowroot.

FRUIT FILLING FOR PIE: Kiwi, Strawberry, Raspberry, etc.

Step 1 WHIZ:

   1 c water (or see p. 85 for some type milk)
   ½ c **date or fruit paste**
   2 tbsp arrowroot

Step 2 Pour into kettle and bring to heat slowly, stirring to keep well mixed until thickened.

Step 3 Remove from heat. Cool.

Step 4 Soften ½ c **real food cheese** or neufchatel, slice **1 large banana,** WHIZ till smooth.

Step 5 Peel and slice **1 c kiwi,** or other fruit.

Step 6 Stir Step 4 into cooled Step 3. Stir in fruit. Pour into **prepared pie shell** of choice. CHILL.

   OPTIONAL: Add 2 or more TB of crushed nutmeats at Step 5. Omit nuts and cheese for (**t**).

MORE CREAM PIES: Strawberry, Kiwi, Papaya, Mango, etc.

Use above methods but use **other** fruits. Fruit may be stirred into batter before cooking (mango) if desired. Delicious if left raw in the filling as with banana.

Note: If fruit adds additional liquid be sure to adjust more arrowroot at 2 tbsp per cup.

HINT: Freeze **1/2 orange** shells to use for dessert fillings.

CREAM CHEESE PIE

Step 1 Beat and Mix or WHIZ:
   12 oz low-fat cream cheese
      (or Real Food yogurt cheese)
   2 whole eggs
   ½ c fruit paste (currant, date or raisin, p. 74)

Step 2 Add **½ tsp vanilla**
   1 cup Real Food sour cream or raw whipping cream

Step 3 Pour into a pie shell.

Step 4 Bake at 350° for about 35 minutes or until baked to center. COOL.

Step 5 Top with glaze of: **Blueberries** or other, see p. 74.

LEMON PIE (*t*)

Step 1 WHIZ in blender:
   2 c pineapple chunks and juice
   ½ c date paste
   4 to 4½ tbsp arrowroot

Step 2 Pour into cooking pot and slowly cook, stirring till thickened.

Step 3 ADD grated rind of **1 lemon and 3 tbsp** of freshly squeezed **lemon juice.**

Step 4 Pour into **baked shell** and allow to tenderize for 24 hours; or pour into **bread-date crust** and SERVE when chilled.

REAL FOOD FAVORITE CAROB PIE (or, use as pudding)

Step 1 WHIZ in blender:
  2 c water or use a milk from page 85
  ½ c chopped warm dates*
  1 tsp vanilla
  4 tbsp arrowroot
  (If water level goes above 2 c add a bit of extra arrowroot . . . 1 tbsp for each ½ c)

Step 2 Pour into cooking pot and slowly bring to heat. Stir to keep smooth while cooking. When filling becomes clear and thick, remove from heat.

Step 3 Mix **3 tbsp carob powder** with 2 tbsp water and add to the Step 2. Stir well and pour into pie shell. COOL.

Step 4 Choose a topping:
  a. Carob flavored glaze from p. 74.
  b. Yogurt-Date cream from p. 75.
  c. **Raw whipping cream** sweetened with date paste. Shred a **carob mint bar** over the top! P. 75.

  *Substitute date paste but allow extra arrowroot for water content of the paste.

DEBI'S DERBY PIE

Step 1 WHIZ: 1 c water (or use a milk from pp 85-87), **2 or 3 eggs,** and **1 c date paste**

Step 2 ADD: ½ c nuts (pecans or walnuts), ½ c unsweetened carob chips

Step 3 STIR and pour into **Nut-Barley or Bread Fruit crust.**

Step 4 BAKE 350° for 30 to 45 min. or until firm. Microwave 30 min. on defrost, turning often.

Step 5 Top with a choice of glazes or use **raw whipping cream sweetened with date paste.** SERVE.

PUMPKIN PIE and variations

WITHOUT NUTS (*t*)
1 c water
½ c cooked rice
1 c date paste
4 tbsp arrowroot
1 tbsp ground coriander
½ tsp salt
Mix well in blender
till very smooth.
ADD 3 c cooked drained
squash or pumpkin

WITH NUTS
1 c water
½ c cashews or nuts
½ c cooked rice
Mix well in blender
till very smooth.
ADD:
1 c date paste
3 cups cooked drained
squash or pumpkin
4 tbsp arrowroot
1 tbsp ground coriander
½ tsp salt

Mix well and pour into a large 10 inch pie shell and bake at 425° for about 15 to 20 minutes, or make two small pies. Let stand for 24 hours to tenderize crust unless using the bread-date crust.

PUMPKIN PIE . . . with eggs

1½ c cooked drained squash or pumpkin
½ c date or fruit paste
2 whole eggs
dash of salt
1 tsp spice
1 c water; or nut milk; or **raw whipping cream**
½ c currants or raisins (optional—may omit)

Combine ingredients. Mix in blender till smooth. Pour into pie shell and bake 425° for 25 minutes or until just set.

A MIXTURE OF SPICE for seasoning desserts:
½ c of coriander to ¼ c anise or cardamon. WHIZ to blend.

A Basic Dough
PIE, CAKE or COOKIE

Step 1 WHIZ till smooth:
   1 c roasted cashews
   ⅔ c water

Step 2 ADD **fruit** for sweeteners and binders:
   i.e.: 1 whole cut up orange (rind and all),
   or: several mashed bananas, or applesauce,
   or: 1 cup fruit; juice, paste or other such.

Step 3 Decide on: pie . . . cake . . . or cookie.

Step 4 Add an **extender:** flour of oats, barley, or wheat.
   i.e.: ½ to 2 cups of flour . . . pie, cake, cookie.

Step 5 Choose: PIE, CAKE, or COOKIE.

"Try Cake"
   Grandmother made a small 2 to 3 inch pan filled with a bit of batter to "test" the cake, pie, or cookie. This is an excellent idea and should be used in Real Food Cooking. Try it!

PIE: Use **Step 1 from Basic Dough. Step 2:** Add the **orange. Step 4:** Add about **1 to 1½ cups of whole wheat flour.** Keep dough fairly smooth and at a consistency that is not too dry.

   ROLL between handiwrap and place in pie pan. Add **filling.** (Cover with another layer if desired) and bake. Or, leave uncovered, with open top. When baked, serve with a **glaze** from page 37.

CAKE: Use **Step 1** from **Basic Dough. Step 2: Fruit juice** and few fruits/vegetables (raisins, grated carrots, etc). Stir in only enough of **Step 4** to make a soft, light cake batter. Bake at 350° in a teflon pan for 45 to 60 minutes, or use microwave in tube pan on defrost. Turn each 5 minutes and rest for 5 minutes. Watch and touch for doneness . . . or make "try cake."

COOKIE: Use **Step 1** from **Basic Dough. Use Step 2.** At **Step 4** add additional items as: **quick rolled oats, currants, raisins, chopped nuts,** chopped **dried fruits, dates,** etc. Then only enough **whole wheat flour** to make a firm batter for drop cookies or rolled cookies. Bake at 350° for about 10 minutes and taste test!

Et Cetera

REAL FOOD FILLED COOKIE

Step 1 Mix ½ **of Basic Dough Recipe, page 45.** Cut in half. Cover to keep moist.

Step 2 Shape one half into a long log on a sheet of waxed paper. Cover with another piece and roll till about 4" wide and 12 to 14" long, and ¼" thick. It will stick to the waxed paper but will pull away.

Step 3 Remove top layer of waxed paper. Spread a layer of **Fruit Paste** (see p. 74, or use dried figs) about ¼" thick down one side of dough. See illustration. Lift paper under dough and carefully lay dough over fig paste. Seal edges, cut away excess to use again. Cut into 2" wedges and lay in baking pan. Repeat with other half of dough.

Step 4 BAKE: Teflon pan, or pan with non-stick. Bake at 350 to 375° for 10 to 15 minutes, until lightly brown. Taste Test, or Try Cake . . . page 45.

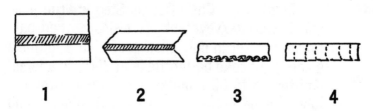

   1   **2**   **3**   **4**

REAL FOOD CANDIES

No. 1 **6 oz unsweetened melted carob chips**
6 to 12 oz Real Food or Neufchatel **cheese**
(the amount of cheese determines the darkness of the candy)
½ cup fruit paste, see page 74

Mix in food processor with blade till well blended and creamed. Pour into square pan lined with handiwrap or waxed paper. Level candy and smooth across top. CHILL till firm.

OPTIONAL:
½ c chopped nuts or currants may be stirred into batter before pouring into pan, or, may be pressed into the top.

No. 2 **¼ cup** roasted powdered **carob**
½ cup Date or Fruit **Paste**

Mix together till well moistened (may add drops of water if needed to mix into smooth paste).

WHIP into **6 or 12 oz of Real Food** or **Neufchatel cheese** or as in No. 1 above.

No. 3 **½ cup** fresh made **peanut butter,** page 75.
4 to 6 oz of **Real Food** or **Neufchatel cheese**
Complete as in No. 1 above.

No. 4 Use any of the above, shape into balls, CHILL, and roll in **nuts,** wheat germ, coconut, melted carob, etc.

NOTE: The amount of cheese determines the amount of darkness desired in the finished candy. The smaller the amount of cheese the darker and stronger the flavor of carob. The larger the amount of cheese the lighter flavored the candy.

CANDY-TYPE SNACKS

Use dried fruits such as slices of apple, pears, banana, apricots, peaches, figs, pitted dates, halves of Mejool dates, and so forth.

Dab a bit of freshly made **peanut butter** into center of **fruit slice** then dip it into grated **coconut,** malt, nuts, or wheat germ.

Put a dab of **Real Food cheese,** Kefir, or Neufchatel cheese on the **fruit.** Eat or dip as shown above.

Work a bit of moistened powdered **carob** into **Real Food Cheese,** Neufchatel, or Kefir and shape into balls. Roll as above.

t Soften **dried fruits** of choice. Then grind or chop very fine. Blend together into logs. Roll and CHILL. Cut off as desired. Roll in finely ground rolled **toasted oat flakes,** barley flakes, or mixed rolled grain flakes which have been finely ground in mill or blender. May also roll the fruit log in Diastatic Malt as found on page 34, for a malty sweet flavor, or roll in finely chopped nuts.

t Soak **wheat berries,** and let sprout. Keep stored in refrigerator. A great chew for snacking. Unsprouted and soaked wheat berries can be used as a gum if chewed till a ball forms. Keep adding more wheat and chewing until a large gum results.

t **Garbanzo** nuts. Soak beans overnight. Let sprout for about one day. Eat as a raw "nut". Or cook until tender, cool. Bake in slow oven till crisp, or bake for 1 hour at 300°. Turn off oven and allow to stay in cooling oven overnight.

Cakes

Create A REAL FOOD FRUIT CAKE

Step 1 MIX 3 cups chopped mixed fruits
1 cup chopped nuts (*t* if omitted)
1 cup fruit paste
1 cup Real Food bread crumbs
2 or 3 eggs (*t* if omitted)
Enough **fruit juice** or liquid to soften mixture.

Step 2 PACK in pan; will not rise if eggs omitted. Bake 350° or microwave on defrost.

Try this one with **little** instruction and be creative!

STRAWBERRY SHORTCAKE (Jiffy)

Step 1 Prepare a Sweet **Bread and Fruit Pie Crust** from page 37.

Step 2 Spread a layer of the Crust into serving plate.

Step 3 Spread a layer of fresh crushed **strawberries** over the layer of crust.

Step 4 Spread a layer of **Cream Topping** of choice or use the Real Rare Treat, page 75.

Step 5 Repeat another layer of crust, fruit and cream. Top with strawberry.

OPTIONAL: Use a slice of Sponge-Angel Cake and layer with strawberries and cream.

REAL FOOD REAL QUICK CAKE (*t* without nuts)

Step 1 Prepare pan: 8 x 8 pan to fit the size of **Real Food or Ezekiel Bread slices**

Step 2 Lay 4 slices on bottom of pan to be sure they fit. Reserve 4 more slices for next layer.

Step 3 Blend all available **fresh or canned fruits** into a sauce in the food blender. Make about **4 cups** sauce. Add apple, banana, date, currant or raisin to sweeten.

Step 4 Bake **walnuts** or **almonds** till browned and crisp. Soften ½ **cup currants** or raisins.

Step 5 ASSEMBLE:
Spread about ½ to ¾ cup of the fruit sauce over bottom of the 8 x 8 pan. Lay in 4 bread slices, over the top of the sauce. Pour additional sauce over the 4 slices of bread. Sprinkle with nuts, currants, or raisins, or all. Repeat another layer of 4 bread slices and pour the remaining sauce over all. (If extra sauce, refrigerate for another meal.)

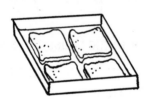

Step 6 Let stand overnight to soak, or bake at once.

Step 7 BAKE: Medium to low oven, 275 to 300° for 1½ to 2 hours. Stores well, and best if sealed with a glaze and left to age for at least 24 hours. To hasten: Cover cake at room temperature with tight lid to steam. Flavors mellow and saturate with age. Store in refrigerator in an airtight pan.

REAL FOOD CAKES

Step 1 Mix and let stand till tender:
1 c quick oat flakes and
1 c HOT water (or use nut milk, p. 85)
(substitute **leftover cereal**)

Step 2 Crush **½ c sesame seed** in blender

Step 3 ADD one of the following:
a. **½ to 1 c softened dates** or date paste
b. **½ c raisins and 1 c pear or applesauce**
c. a like combination or substitute

Step 4 **3 to 6 eggs,** well beaten.

Step 5 **Whole wheat flour, barley flour, rice flour, or etc.,**
½ to 1 cup to form a soft firm cake-like batter.

Step 6 BAKE: Pour into teflon pan or pan prepared with non-stick and sprinkled with cornmeal or coarse flour. Bake 350° for 45 to 60 minutes or until sides are free. Bake on defrost in microwave glass tube pan for 40 minutes. Waiting 5 minutes between each turn at 10-minute intervals.

SUGGESTIONS AND CHANGES:
Nuts and dried fruits may be added.
Grated zucchini, carrot, etc., may be added.
Additional fruits and fruit juices mean more cooking time, and a change in flour addition. Make a "Try Cake."
May omit eggs altogether! (t)
Be creative.
Improves with age as they mellow in refrigeration!
½ to 1 c of raw whipping cream is acceptable to substitute for nuts or natural fat in any cake recipe.

REAL FOOD FRUIT-CUSTARD CAKE

Step 1 PREPARE:

½ **cup** each   whole or slivered **almonds**
softened **currants** or raisins
dates cut small
cut dried **figs** or **other fruit**
walnuts, whole or sliced

or PREPARE:
½ **cup** whole/slivered **almonds**
½ **cup walnuts,** whole or sliced
2 cups chopped **mixed dried fruits**

Step 2 ⅓ **cup brazil** nuts blended until smooth
(may substitute cashew nuts)

Step 3 ¼ **c rolled baby oats**
(or leftover breakfast cereal)

Step 4 Mix blended nuts with baby oats in food blender.

Step 5 ADD:
2 to 4 whole eggs
2 whole bananas added for sweetening
1 tsp vanilla
1 tsp coriander/anise mix
¼ **tsp salt**
TURN ON BLENDER and mix till well blended.

Step 6 Pour over fruits from Step 1.

Step 7 Add ½ to 1 c **Real Food Bread Crumbs** and stir till batter is like a light custard. Additional **fruit juice** or water may be added for right consistency.

Step 8 BAKE: Pour into prepared microwave tube pan and bake at defrost 35 to 45 minutes, turning each 10 minutes and allowing a 5-minute rest. Cake will fall from sides of pan when done. Conventional oven 350° for 45 to 60 minutes or falls from sides of pan.

REAL FOOD SPONGE — ANGEL CAKE

Step 1 Pour **1 c egg whites** into bowl and whip until frothy.

Step 2 ADD ¾ **c soft smooth date paste,** p. 74, and continue beating until soft peaks form.

Step 3 Add flavoring and **salt** as desired.

Step 4 Fold in ¾ **c fine barley flour** (or may use rice flour or whole wheat if it is sifted several times to make fine)!

Step 5 BAKE: Pour into 4 c or 1 quart teflon pan, or clean dry pan, 350° for 30 to 40 minutes.

> **OPTIONAL:** Before pouring into the pan try adding 1/4 c unsweetened carob chips, a few finely chopped nuts, or ¼ c dry currants finely dusted with barley flour.

REAL FOOD SPONGE — Rice Flour and Egg Cake

Step 1 Pour **1 c yolks** or mixed egg yolks and whites into food processor (5 to 6 **eggs**)
ADD:
½ **c soft currants** or raisins
¼ **c date paste**
salt as desired

Step 2 Pulsate till blended and all fruits dissolved into batter.

Step 3 ADD **1-1¼ c rice flour** (or barley or other) and pulsate only until mixed
ADD **1 tsp vanilla**

Step 4 Pour into 6 c or 1½ quart teflon baking pan

Step 5 BAKE in moderate oven 350° for 30 to 40 minutes (or "Try Cake," p. 45).

> **OPTIONAL:** Before baking, drop a few pieces of unsweetened carob chips into batter and carefully fold in; or add additional nuts, chopped fruits, or currants.

EVERYDAY REAL FOOD CAKE (*t* without nuts)

Step 1 6 to 8 slices **REAL FOOD** or Ezekial-type bread. Blend to soft crumbs.

Step 2 ½ to ¾ **c softened dates** or date paste or substitute: ½ c condensed unsweetened apple juice, apple sauce or other sweetener.

Step 3 ½ **c softened raisins** (or chopped dried fruits) ¼ **c chopped or whole nutmeats** (optional)

Step 4 Mix bread crumbs with fruits. Stir well, or mix in food processor till blended. Add any additional fruit juice or liquid to form a soft batter. In baking, the bread crumbs and fruits will absorb lots of the liquid. Pack in pan (will not rise).

Step 5 Bake. Pour into pan covered with non-stick or a teflon baking pan. Bake slowly to bring out flavors and not overbake (250 to 300° for 45 minutes to 2 hrs.). More fruits mean more cooking. Trial and error will help you develop your own cake.

Step 6 REST CAKE in refrigerator for a day or so. Cake improves with age. Also use a **glaze or topping.** See p. 74-75.

Step 7 MICROWAVE: In glass tube pan on defrost for 45 minutes to 1 hour or more. Turn and rest at 15 minute intervals.

MERINGUE FOR PIE TOPPING OR COOKIE

2 to 3 whites of egg, beaten until frothy.
ADD **2 to 3 tbsp of date paste.**
WHIP until stiff.
   Spread over pie and bake 300° till lightly brown.
OR: ADD choice of: 1 c **nutmeats,** 1 c **currants,** or **coconut,** or **carob chips.** DROP on no-stick sheet by spoonful and bake as above, 300°.

DINNER ENTREES

Dinner Entrees

SAMPLE VEGETABLE PLATE (*t*)

Purchase and prepare:

Fresh **Asparagus** spears 3 to 4 inches long. Reserve edible remainder for another meal.

Small whole **carrots** or carefully quartered, allowing 5 pieces for each serving.

1 large **cauliflower** section for each serving

1 large or 3 to 5 smaller **mushrooms** each

½" slice of large **onion** for each serving

1 thick slice of large peeled **tomato,** 1" thick for each serving **(breaded)**

1 section **broccoli** for each serving

SAUTE: in ¼ c water one slice of **onion** for each serving. Cook slowly (covered) until tender. Thicken the liquid into **Onion Glaze** (No. 3, p. 88).

STEAM in small amount of water until tender:

... carrots in pan by themselves to reserve the liquid for glaze, see p. 88.

... cauliflower until tender. Prepare sauce as described on p. 88, No. 2.

... broccoli until tender, keeping good green color.

... mushrooms in small amount of water. Reserve liquid for glaze. Season with lemon juice.

... steam asparagus spears only until tender; takes very little time.

BROIL

... the tomato and sprinkle with seasoned bread crumbs, (see p. 88).

SERVE:

Place tomato in center of serving plates. Arrange the complementary vegetables around the tomato. Try keeping colors attractive. Pour each individual sauce over its own vegetable. Put mushrooms next to asparagus for lemon to mix.

SERVE each plate individually arranged, or serve from common center Chop Plate, allowing each diner to serve himself.

OPTIONALS:

Serve seasonal vegetables such as: **snap peas, zucchini, green beans, shredded cabbage,** etc.

CHICKEN AND/OR RICE CASSEROLE (*t* if meat omitted)

FAST . . . 10 minutes to fix

SAUTE: 8 to 10 mushrooms in tbsp water. Stir in teflon pan till tender. Set aside. Cover.

SAUTE: ½ c chopped onion in same manner.

MEANWHILE:
Prepare vegetables: Thaw or cook ½ to ¾ cup Okra, bell pepper, frozen peas, carrots, and/or other vegetables. Use mixed vegetables, or all same kind.

DEFROST: 1 to 2 cups cooked natural rice.

MIX: Dump vegetables onto rice, add onions and mushrooms. Add herbs to taste. Season with garlic chips or powder, salt to taste, or use fresh sea kelp. Add water for moisture as needed.

MICROWAVE: Reheat for 3 to 4 minutes or until warmed throughout.

OPTIONALS: Use: ½ cup nuts of choice
½ to 1 c chopped poultry or fish
Cover top with seasoned Bread Crumbs.

CORN SOUFFLE (*t*) (For using Garden Vegetable in a loaf)

ASSEMBLE   1½ c fresh corn off the cob
IN FOOD   1 small summer squash
BLENDER: 1 medium carrot
            ½ c peeled egg plant
            ¼ c sweet onion
            ¼ green sweet pepper
            ½ cup fresh mashed tomato

WHIZ: and blend till smooth. Pour into casserole. Top with ¼ c seasoned breadcrumbs. Bake for 30 to 40 minutes at 350°. Microwave in covered casserole, on low heat, 30 to 40 minutes. Test.

GRAPE LEAF ROLL (*t*)

Step 1 Harvest **fresh young grape leaves** in the spring. Choose those toward the end of the vine, which are the newest.

Step 2 Lay a leaf on kitchen work board and place about 1 tbsp of **"filler"*** in the center of the leaf and "roll" leaf around the filler. If a second leaf is needed to hold the filling in the leaf, wrap it around as well.

Step 3 Lay the filled leaves on the bottom of a flat baking dish.

Step 4 Pour a seasoned **sauce as on p. 67** over the leaves; then place a saucer over the leaves to hold them down into the sauce. Cover with a lid.

Step 5 Bake or simmer about an hour or until tender. Taste test the first time.

*Filler Use seasoned **rice,** seasoned **bulgar,** or whatever left over grain or legume as desired. **Chicken** may be used in addition. Season with **cumin** for a near eastern flavor.

YEAR 'ROUND FRESH GARDEN MEDLEY (*t*)

Original every time: Inventory garden and refrigerator. Select 3 above ground vegetables to each below ground. Wash and scrub to remove dirt and unseen molds.

Step 1 SLICE or CUBE into cooking pot in order: **Onion** or **leek, string beans, carrots celery, potato, green pepper, summer squashes,** (greens) **parsley,** and slices of **tomato** over top.

Step 2 ADD ¼ c **water,** cover and place over controlled heat. Do not overcook, or let color change. EAT at once.

Pilaff (Near East Favorites)

RICE (t)

SAUTE: ½ c chopped onion in 2 tbsp water; add 2 mashed cloves of garlic; and one 4 oz. can of mushrooms. Herbs to taste. Use ¼ tsp ground cumin and ¼ tsp cumin seed as well as lemon thyme, oregano, etc.

ADD: 1 c Dextrinized brown natural rice and enough water (liquid or broth) to cover by 1 inch. Bring to a soft simmer boil, reduce heat and keep warm till all water is absorbed. (Add more liquid if necessary). For eastern texture, add 1" pieces of vermicilli for texture. May use liquid of Chicken broth. When tender, SERVE.

BARLEY (t)

SAUTE: ½ c chopped onion in 2 tbsp water, add 2 mashed garlic cloves, and 1 c sliced fresh mushrooms, and herbs to taste.

ADD: 1 cup dextrinized pearl barley. (See p. 34) Cover with at least 2 c water (or broth) and bake in a S L O W oven at 300 to 325°. Cook S L O W L Y and turn carefully several times while baking, not to disturb the texture of the barley. COVER. Each ½ hour open oven, take off lid and keep a watch on water level. Add liquid as it is being absorbed. Will take about 2 hours of slow baking.

OPTIONAL:
Use other whole dextrinized grains in the same manner.
Sprinkle with almonds or other nuts.
Add chopped parsley to trim.

BLACK BEANS and RICE From Cuba (*t*)

SOAK: 2c water and **1c or 6 oz. black beans.** Soak over-night, or heat water and beans to boiling and boil 3 to 4 minutes. Turn off heat, cover and let stand for 1 hour.

SAUTE: (in 2 tbsp water) **1 small onion,** sliced; **1 small chopped green pepper; 2 mashed garlic cloves; 1 bay leaf; dried oregano leaves; ½ tsp. cumin,** and a sprinkle of whole **cumin seed;** salt as desired.

ADD: to beans, stir well, and enough water additionally to cover beans if needed. Heat to full simmer and cook for about two hours, until beans are tender and most liquid absorbed.

SERVE: over **hot brown rice,** accompanied with a green **tossed salad, hot bread,** or rolls.

REAL FOOD EGGPLANT (*t*)

Step 1 Prepare **eggplant.** Hasten by partially prebaking in microwave. Slice without peeling into 1" slices.

Step 2 Lay into baking dish in a single layer.

Step 3 Top with some seasoned or plain **bread crumbs.** Spread generously with **REAL FOOD** tomato sauce, using extra herbs such as **oregano and cumin.**

Step 4 Bake 350° for 30 to 45 minutes, or until tender. Excellent rewarmed.

Alternate: Cut precooked eggplant into cubes; add toasted cubes of sea-soned or plain bread. Stir and bake in small patties in crock oven, open non-stick skillet, or conventional oven till tender. Taste test.

CHILI RELLENO serves 2

Step 1 Prepare **2 whole seeded and peeled green chili.** Use fresh roasted or canned.

Step 2 Prepare **2 tbsp Real Food Firm Pimiento Yogurt Cheese.**

Step 3 Whip **1 egg white** until firm.

Step 4 Dry the chili with paper towel and stuff with 1 tbsp of the cheese.

Step 5 BAKE: Lay ¼ of the beaten egg white in a teflon frying pan in the shape of the chili. Lay one stuffed chili on top. Repeat with remaining chili. Cover both chili with the remaining egg white and shape over and around each chili.

Bake S L O W L Y in pan until golden brown on under side. Turn and repeat on all sides. Do not overheat the soft cheese inside as it will toughen. Serve at once. Salt and season to taste.

Optional: Use the Real Food Crepe Batter as a covering for the chili in place of the egg white. Cook over low heat.

REAL FOOD BREAD DRESSING (t)
For stuffing fowl or use as side dish

WHIZ **4 to 6 slices sprouted grain or Real Food Bread**

ADD **½ c finely sliced or cubed celery**
¼ c chopped parsley
¼ c chopped onion
2 cloves chopped garlic
¼ to ½ c currents or raisins
¼ c raw cranberries (fresh or frozen)
Herbs to taste or use "Herb Mix" p. 69.

MIX and BAKE in covered dish 30 to 45 minutes at 350°. Taste test. Or use to stuff a Chicken or a Turkey.

FINGER TAMALE (*t* by adjusting the filling)

Step 1 THE SAUCE. Sauté **1 small chopped onion** with **½ chopped sweet green pepper** in small amount of water. **Herbs** to taste. Add **16 oz. drained whole tomatoes** which have been sieved or processed. Simmer, or use Real Food Tomato Sauce from p. 67.

Step 2 THE DOUGH. Blend **1 cup Masa Harina** (dehydrated masa flour) with ¼ c warm water mixed with ¼ to ⅓ cup of above sauce, and any additional seasoning to taste. Flavor and texture of the dough determines the tamale. Mix into a pliable ball, cover, and let stand while preparing corn husk.

Step 3 THE HUSK. Soak about **6 to 8 large wide corn husks in hot water.** When pliable, drain and wipe dry.

Step 4 THE FILLING. 1 tbsp thickened sauce from above. **1 tsp firm yogurt cheese, an olive, some vegetable, ie: steamed carrot slice, 1 tsp mashed beans, chip of green chili pepper, cube of chicken breast,** etc.

Step 5 ASSEMBLE. Lay a large corn husk on the working table; with spatula spread about 1 to 2 tbsp of the soft dough over the bottom, wider section of the corn husk. (If dough seems too stiff, thin with a bit more sauce or water). One half of the corn husk should be covered (see illustration). Drop 1 tbsp of the thickened sauce in the center of the dough-covered husk; lay an olive in the center, one tsp of the yogurt cheese, choice of a vegetable, and a few pieces of green chili. ROLL the corn husk, long side to long side, sealing the sauce in the center. Fold the small top down over the dough section to keep the sauce inside.

Step 6 Place the Tamale in a steamer with the folded side DOWN and the two open sides up to keep sauce in the tamale!

(A ½ brick or rock in the center of a large kettle will keep the tamale in place while steaming). Continue until all dough is used up. Will make 6 to 8 tamales, depending upon the size of the corn husks.

Step 7 STEAM for about an hour. Serve. Or COOL and refrigerate and resteam. Excellent when resteamed!

REAL FOOD ENCHILADAS (*t* by adjusting the filling)

Step 1 Prepare basic **REAL FOOD Tomato Sauce.** Change seasoning by adding **diced green chili, cumin,** or use package of dry Enchilada seasoning.

Step 2 Warm and prepare **Corn Tortilla** for wrapping. Each tortilla can be reheated on both sides in a teflon pan.

Step 3 Dip warmed tortilla in the sauce to dampen, or, spread sauce on both sides with a brush.

Step 4 Place 1 to 2 tbsp of a **filling** into the center of tortilla, (see filling below). Roll, starting at one side of the circle. Lift carefully and place the loose side of the tortilla down in a square or oblong baking dish. Repeat till dish is filled.

Step 5 Cover with remaining sauce, sprinkle finely chopped onion, parsley and green pepper over all. BAKE 350° for 15 to 20 minutes, or until heated throughout. Serve at once.

FILLING: Cooked **mashed beans, 1 tbsp of pimiento-yogurt,** an **olive,** or **cube of fat-free skinned chicken.** OR mashed **legumes** of any kind, chopped bell pepper, etc.

Real Food Ravioli

DOUGH

Step 1 MIX together and KNEAD
3 c whole wheat or barley flour
3 whole eggs
½ c liquid   ½ tsp salt if desired

Step 2 Cover and let rest.

REAL FOOD SAUCE

See page 67. MIX and let simmer.

REAL FOOD RAVIOLI FILLING

Step 1 MIX well and let stand for flavors to marinate, (or mix day ahead and refrigerate).

1 c chopped cooked greens
1½ c firm yogurt cheese (see page 83-84)
1-2 c finely ground REAL FOOD bread crumbs or
1 c cold water crackers, finely ground
2 large mashed garlic cloves
(optional) **2 whole beaten eggs and salt.**
(Adjust amount of bread crumbs for a firm but not DRY filling)

ASSEMBLE

Step 1 DIVIDE **DOUGH** into equal portions. Roll out one portion, using flour very sparingly. Roll dough until it is quite thin . . . 1/16". Do not tear the dough! Turn frequently. Roll dough in circle or in an oblong rectangle.

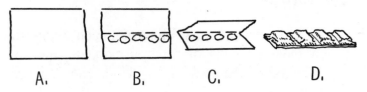

A.   B.   C.   D.

Step 2 CUT rectangle into strips 2 to 3 inches wide and as long as possible. Each strip to be folded in half once (longways), the circle folded in half once.

Step 3 DROP 1 tsp **RAVIOLI FILLING** along the edge of the 3″ wide strip, spacing about 1½ to 2″ apart. See illustrations A and B.

Step 4 When finished, ½ of the strip will be filled. Use damp brush and lightly dampen empty half with water.

Step 5 FOLD, Lift empty half of strip over the filled strip. See illustration C. Gently press dough together between mounds of filling to form a bond around the mounds of filling. See illustration D. With the edge of an old-fashioned yardstick, firmly press the dough together to form a good bond.

Step 6 CUT and separate each pillow with a pastry cutter or knife. Using tines of a fork, reinforce the edges of each pillow to form an individual ravioli. REPEAT.

Step 7 Use same process for a large circle of dough by lifting half of the dough over the other half of the large circle.

Step 8 Set pillows of dough aside on a flat surface, sprinkled with **rice flour,** or a coase flour to prevent sticking. (May freeze and repack into bags.) COOK to use at once.

Step 9 BOILING: Fill large pot with water, bring to boil. Drop each ravioli, one at a time into moving water. Cook gently until tender. (Taste test). Type of flour used will determine the cooking time.

Step 10 DRAIN carefully and layer with **SAUCE,** (and **REAL FOOD** cheese or cheese filling if desired) in a baking dish.

Step 11 Reheat gently to serve without overheating the cheese. 350° for 15 to 20 minutes. Reduce heat and barely simmer till ready to serve.

LASAGNA

Step 1 BOIL **Whole Wheat,** Sesame, or a Vegetable Lasagna **noodle** until tender. Drain. Lay separate so none touch each other, and cover with a damp cloth. Or, may store in cool water until ready to use, then drain and dry.

Step 2 ASSEMBLE
Real Food Cheese Filling, page 84.

Real Food Tomato Sauce, page 67.
An oven casserole wide enough for either a double, or a single stack of Noodles.

Step 3 Cover bottom of casserole dish with some of the tomato sauce.

Lay one layer of noodles and then spread with a layer of REAL FOOD cheese filling followed with a layer of sauce. Repeat. If casserole is deep enough, make up to 4 to 6 layers. Many layers makes for a more colorful display when served. Top layer should be the sauce.

Step 4 BAKE at 350° for 15 to 30 minutes. Simmer till served. Do not OVERHEAT the cheese. Soft yogurt cheese will toughen with heat.

Step 5 Cut in generous wedge as wide as the noodle and about 3 to 4 inches long. Lift carefully and as it sets on serving plate allow the many layers to barely tip for a nice display. Sprinkle with **parsley.**

SPAGHETTI (*t*)

Boil **whole wheat,** sesame or any vegetable **spaghetti** until tender. Drain and spoon onto serving plate. Top with **sauce,** and serve with toasted strips of Real Food Bread and garlic salt.

QUICKIE RAVIOLI or LASAGNA

Step 1 Use the **DOUGH** (p. 64). Roll into strips. Cut narrow strips 1" or 2" at most.

Step 2 Drop into boiling water until tender.

Step 3 Layer dough alternately with **fillings** and **sauce** into casserole.

Step 4 Bake 350° for 15 to 20 minutes. SERVE.

REAL FOOD TOMATO SAUCE for Spaghetti, Lasagna, etc.

Step 1 Sauté **2 large chopped red sweet onions** in small amount of water.

Step 2 Add

1½ to 2 qts. whole tomatoes (put through a sieve or process in machine till mashed)
2 large mashed garlic cloves
2 stalks, leaves and all of chopped celery
2 large sweet carrots (shredded)
2 large sweet carrots (finely grated)
½ c chopped parsley
8 to 16 oz. fresh sliced or canned mushrooms
1 green or red sweet pepper, chopped

Seasonings to taste: or 1 tbsp ea. basil, marjoram, oregano, golden thyme, ¼ tsp rosemary, sage, etc.
Optional: ½ c sliced olives
½ c chopped garbanzo beans

Step 3 Cook in large kettle for several hours at a steady simmer. Long slow cooking enhances the flavor.

Step 4 For a thicker sauce if too thin: Add a bit of **whole wheat flour** moistened with a bit of water and stir into sauce until desired thickness is obtained.

Note: If excess sauce is left over from whatever recipe is being made, Freeze it in 1 c containers for future use. Defrosts quickly!

A BASIC LOAF (Original every time)
(*t* by adjusting optionals)

Step 1 SAUTE **onion** in ¼ c water

Step 2 ADD remaining vegetables from No. 1 below. Steam slightly. WHIZ all in blender.

Step 3 Select from No. 2 below. If using Garbanzos or beans puree ¾ of them in blender. If using corn, puree all of it. If additional liquid is needed for blades to work in the blender, add fresh tomato or water.

Step 4 Pour blender Mix from Step 2 into the 2 c of grain or legume from Step 3 which has been cooked in advance until tender. ADD any of the optionals under No. 3 below, and top with **seasoned bread crumbs.** BAKE 350° 30 to 45 minutes.

No. 1 Vegetables ½ c diced sweet onions
1½ c ½ c green chopped pepper
¼ c chopped celery
¼ c choice: carrot, eggplant, summer
   squash, etc.
1 mashed garlic clove

No. 2 Precooked a. 1 c Garbanzo, lentil, corn, etc.
2 c b. 1 c bulgar, rolled oats, barley, etc.
OR use 2 cups a; or 2 cups b or 1 cup each.

No. 3 Optionals 1 peeled tomato ¼ c nutmeats
½ c parsley ¼ c drained olives
½ c sliced mushrooms
½ c skinned cooked cubed chicken
½ c cooked cubed lamb
½ to 1 c breadcrumbs
¼ to ½ c leftover vegetable sauce

STUFFED CABBAGE LEAVES (*t*)

Step 1 Select **4 to 6 large outside cabbage leaves** (if difficult to remove drop whole cabbage into large kettle of boiling water until softened). Cut out core to make lifting the leaves easier.

Step 2 Simmer leaves in kettle of water until pliable and transparent. Do not overcook.

Step 3 Prepare filling: Use leftovers of **vegetable** and **grain dishes** or use **rice, pilaff, lentil dishes, bean dishes,** etc. Season to taste.

Step 4 Dry the leaf with cloth. Lay leaf on working surface. If core of leaf is heavy, cut it out as shown in illustration a. Lay ¼ to ½ cup of filling in center of leaf and fold over sides to cover, and roll securely to hold filling in. Turn upside down into baking dish. Repeat until dish is filled.

Step 5 Cover the cabbage leaves with a baking sauce such as the **Tomato Sauce** used for spaghetti and lasagna on page 67.

Step 6 Bake: 350° for 30 to 40 minutes, or until tender and well heated. Serve.

a   cut core out of leaf

A MIXTURE OF HERBS for seasoning vegetables:
WHIZ in blender till smooth.
1 tbsp each:
   Dried **kelp, oregano, basil, lemon thyme, parsley, garlic and onion powder**
1 tsp of dried **rosemary**, a few dried garlic chips
Vary amounts of each herb. Add any additional herbs desired. **For lamb, chicken,** and **meats** add some dried **sage** leaves and dried **mint** leaves.

Joanne & George's PIEROGIs (German-Balkin)

Step 1 **2 c flour** (wheat, barley, or etc.)
1 egg (slightly beaten)
½ c lukewarm water
¼ tsp salt

Step 2 Mix all ingredients and knead until dough is soft and well formed.

Step 3 Roll out on board as thin as possible and cut into circles or squares about 2 to 3″ across.

Step 4 Place one tbsp of **filling** (below; see illustration a.) into each circle. Fold over and wet edges and pinch to seal (see illustration b.). Be sure it is well sealed.

Step 5 Drop into moving boiling water and cook until pierogi rises to the top and (taste test) for doneness. Remove and cut open.
Remove with slotted spoon so as to drain.

Step 6 Make glaze to cover. See choices below:

Glaze: 1. Use the **vegetable sauce** mix on p. 88 but thinned a bit more.
2. Use **arrowroot** base glaze, seasoned to taste with mushrooms, and or sautéed onions, etc.
3. Use fresh raw sweet butter, or a small amount of olive oil.

Filling: 1. **Dry curd cottage cheese**
2. **Mashed potatoes**
3. **Real Food yogurt cheese**
4. **Home-canned or fresh sauerkraut**

REAL FOOD ORIENTAL DELIGHT (t if nuts omitted)
Designed to use up kitchen and garden vegetables

Step 1 Prepare:
1 c julienne carrot strips
1 c small branches broccoli
1 c snap peas or ½ c frozen peas
½ to 1 c sliced fresh mushrooms
    or a 4 to 6 oz. can
½ c chopped green garden onions
1 green or red sweet pepper, cut in long wide strips
Bamboo shoots or other oriental favorite
1 large mashed garlic clove.

Optionals: ½ c peeled toasted almonds
           1 c bean or other sprouts
           1 c or more other vegetables
           1 c steamed rice (stirred in)

Step 2 Sauté onion in 2 tbsp water; add fresh vegetables, sauté, then add any optional choices. Steam over low heat only until tender. Do not allow the color of the vegetables to change. (Add frozen peas last with the glaze).

Step 3 **Glaze.** Pour the liquid into sauce pan. Add arrowroot to make thinnish sauce; see page 74. ½ c liquid to 1 tsp arrowroot. Add seasonings of choice: soya mineral, soya sauce, teriyaki sauce, kitchen bouquet, or herbs to taste. Return to vegetables and stir for glaze.

Step 4 Serve plain, or over **steamed rice, bean threads, noodles,** or other grains.

71

REAL FOOD PONSET (Malaya-Philippines)
(*t* if meat omitted)

Step 1 Prepare ingredients:
  ½ lb. **Rice Stick** (found in Specialty stores)
  1 large chopped sweet onion
  2 large mashed garlic cloves
  2 c sliced fresh or 1 8 oz. can mushrooms
  1 cup sliced celery
  2 c sliced cabbage (napa type if available)
  Optional: 1 c cooked cubed chicken and/or fish

Step 2 Soak the Rice Stick in very hot water

Step 3 Sauté onion in 1 tbsp of water, add cabbage, celery, garlic and mushrooms. Add seasonings to taste. Soy sauce, etc.

Step 4 When vegetables are tender. Add the soaked and drained Rice Sticks. Simmer and add additional seasonings to taste.

Step 5 Serve with fresh **hot bread** and **lemon wedges.**

BAKED POTATO CHIPS (Use sweet, yams, or white potato)
(*t*)

Step 1 Cut the potato into large wedges. Cut longwise on the potato and make generous wedges at least ½ inch or more thick.

Step 2 Bake in a convection or traditional oven until brown and tender. 450°. Serve with soups, or vegetable dishes, or as a snack for dips.

Sauces and Toppings for Desserts

In these recipes adjust liquid to create desired consistency of sauce or topping. Increase liquid for a thinner paste and decrease liquid for a thicker paste.

REAL FOOD FRUIT PASTE (used for sweetening)

1 c seeded dates
½ c liquid (water or fruit juice)

COMBINE water and dates. Place over heat or in a microwave to slightly soften. WHIZ in blender. Stop to push sides down. WHIZ again. Adjust thickness with additional liquid.

BASIC MIXING INSTRUCTIONS for Arrowroot

t 2 tbsp per 1 cup liquid for a THICK sauce
1 tbsp per 1 cup liquid for THIN pouring sauce
(a very QUICK cooking thickening agent)

> ...PREMIX arrowroot with cold water, or LIGHTLY sprinkle into hot water, but stir constantly to prevent lumping.
> ...Re-heating of arrowroot will thin sauce.
> ...Cook or heat only until sauce is clear; cooks instantly, no need to boil away.
> ...Substitute for cornstarch or tapioca.

REAL FOOD (low-fat) FRUIT TOPPING

1 c Real Food Yogurt and 2 tbsp Fruit Paste
If WHIZZED in blender will become liquid and pour
If STIRRED by **hand** will stay thick.

> Use other fruits for paste such as banana, berries, etc.

REAL FOOD QUICK 'n EASY CAKE & PIE GLAZE

t MIX ¾ c fruit juice (or water) with **2 tbsp arrowroot powder.** COOK over medium heat, stirring constantly till comes to low boil or turns clear, about one minute. Remove from heat. ADD ¼ c **unsweetened frozen orange juice,** or other frozen unsweetened concentrate, or fresh whole fruit to flavor. (Allow for additional liquid in fresh fruit.)

WHIPPED APPLE/NUT TOPPING — Cream

Step 1 Grind in nut grinder or WHIZ till smooth in dry food blender, **1 cup raw cashews.**

Step 2 Core but do not peel **2** golden delicious **apples.**
Add **¼ to ⅓ cup** unsweetened frozen **apple juice,** or just enough to get blender working.
WHIZ in food blender, pushing down to keep going.
ADD **1 tsp lemon juice.**
Whiz till smooth.

Step 3 ADD the ground cashews to the blended apple mix.
Blend until smooth. Will resemble whipped cream.
Use as parfait with fruits or as topping for salads of fruit or for the topping on pie or cake.

REAL FOOD SUNDAE, OR SAUCE (*t* if nuts omitted)

Mix in blender, or in bowl by hand:
2 tbsp Toasted Carob powder and **2 tbsp Date** or **Fruit Paste.** Add enough HOT water to make a smooth sauce or glaze.
Try glazing a frozen **banana . . .** then DIP in chopped **nuts.**

FRESH REAL FOOD PEANUT BUTTER

Step 1 Purchase the **nuts** which are dry roasted and ready for grinding in a commercial machine, oven-dry, or raw peanuts (Legume).

Step 2 WHIZ ½ to 1 cup nuts in processor until smooth.
Will start to form a ball then become a smooth liquid.

Once in a while... Special Treats

REAL FOOD PEANUT TOPPING
>**6 oz Real Food Cheese** (Kefir or Neufchatel)
>**3 to 6 oz** fresh ground **peanut butter**
>WHIZ in food processor or blender until smooth.
>Good for topping on pie, cake, or cookies.

REAL FOOD BASIC CREAM CHEESE TOPPING
>**6 oz Real Food Cheese** (Kefir or Neufchatel)
>**¼ cup Fruit Paste**
>WHIZ in food processor or blender until smooth.
>Good for topping on pie, cake, or cookies

REAL FOOD CREAM CHEESE TOPPING with fresh fruits
>**6 to 12 oz Real Food Cheese** (Kefir or Neufchatel)
>**1 to 1½ cups fresh fruit** of choice:
>Kiwi
>Banana
>Papaya
>Peach
>Strawberry
>etc.
>WHIZ in food processor or blender until smooth.
>RICH and DELICIOUS. Used all kinds of ways!

REAL SPECIAL TREAT
>**½ pint Raw Whipping Cream**
>Whip, adding
>**¼ to ¾ cup date or fruit paste**
>**Vanilla** to taste
>Serve as topping on carob pie, or freeze for frozen ice cream.
>ALTERNATE: Crush ½ to ¾ c fresh fruits and fold through. Serve or freeze.

Salad Dressings, etc.

Use the following suggestions with **1 cup of Real Food Yogurt** or a non-fat yogurt with 1 g or less per cup. Some of the dressing suggestions do not need yogurt added at all.

Yogurt will be THIN if seasoning is WHIZZED in with food blender . . . and will stay thicker if only stirred in with a mixing stick, by hand.

1. To Yogurt add **1 tbsp lemon juice, ½ tsp dry minced garlic, 1 tsp dry minced onion,** choice of seeds, such as **dill, cumin, celery,** etc.

2. **1 tbsp lemon juice, ½ of a fresh cuke, ¼ tsp garlic powder, ½ to 1 tsp salad herbs.** Blend well in machine. Add yogurt.

3. Mix in blender: **1 whole peeled tomato, ½ c sweet onion, 1 large garlic clove, 1 tbsp lemon juice, basil,** and **herbs** to taste. WHIZ. Use with or without yogurt.

4. Blend any of the **fruit pastes,** p. 74, into the yogurts in amount desired, i.e., 2 tbsp to 1 c, or taste test, or whiz a bit of fresh fruit and stir into yogurt to taste. Fresh banana whizzed till smooth, an apple, or an orange. Try some unsweetened dried coconut stirred into yogurt.

5. CREATE: WHIZ in blender 1 cup of whatever is being
t   mixed into salad: **Lettuce, onion, pepper, cuke, tomato,** etc. Blend until liquid, add some **lemon juice** and **herbs,** and use as a fresh dressing! EXCELLENT and HANDY TO USE FOR SCRAPS!

6. **½ c lemon juice** and **¼ c water.** ADD **¼ tsp garlic pow-**
t   **der, ¼ tsp dry chopped onion, ½ tsp herbs.** Mix to taste. (For purchased mix . . . read label and be sure no oils are added, as well as no honey, or sugars.) Shake or stir and let stand till ready to use. Sprinkle over salads.

7. Base for dressing: Heat ½ c water with **1 tbsp arrowroot,**
t stirring until clear. Cool. Add any of the before mentioned herbs or suggestions. Season to taste.

8. Base for dressing: Heat 1 c water and **1 tbsp flax seed.**
t Cook about 5 minutes. Blend and strain. Season as in 7 above.

9. Mix and blend well: **½ c fresh lemon juice** with 3 or more
t peeled large **garlic** cloves. Add pinch of fresh **tarragon** or basil for flavor. Chill in shaker bottle and keep in refrigerator for quick use.

10. FIESTA SALAD DRESSING:
t **1 16 oz jar whole drained tomatoes**
2 fresh peeled ripe tomatoes, sliced and chopped
1 red sweet spanish onion, finely chopped
1 tbsp diced green chili (optional)
1 tsp fresh lemon juice
1 tsp basil or fresh basil leaves
    Pinch of additional herbs to taste: lemon thyme, etc.

WHIZ the whole tomato with blades, or press through a sieve. Mix well with remaining vegetables, or may process quickly on PULSE for 2 seconds. Chill.

11. CREAMY FIESTA DRESSING:
Stir **1 c of Fiesta** into **½ c yogurt cheese.** Chill.

12. YOGURT AND CUKE DRINK OR DRESSING
WHIZ in blender until smooth: **1 c yogurt** and **1 whole fresh garden cuke,** skin and all. Chill and drink.

13. REAL FOOD CHEESE SPREAD (especially for pizza)
½ c sour cream from p. 79 or Real Food Yogurt Cheese from p. 82. **1 tbsp chopped pimiento.** Mix together in blender until smooth.

14. REAL FOOD MEXICAN SPREAD
½ c **sour cream,** or Real Food Yogurt Cheese
2 tsp diced green chili
Mix well together in blender until smooth, or stir to blend.

15. DIPS — DIPS — DIPS
See preceding pages for ideas. Blend **avocado** with **lemon juice.** Blend fresh vegetables and add to one of the bases; add **herbs** and **seeds** to one of the bases. ADD **DRIED ONION FLAKES** to thicken up a loose dip and chill overnight. Create a dip! **Dill** seeds are excellent!

16. QUICK KETCHUP
t **1 c tomato paste**
1 tbsp thick fruit paste, p. 74
¼ tsp salt
2 tbsp fresh lemon juice
¼ tsp onion powder
½ tsp garlic powder
½ tsp paprika
½ tsp herbs to taste: basil, etc.
MIX with whip till smooth. Refrigerate.

17. REAL FOOD SOUR CREAM
Step 1 1 c REAL FOOD Yogurt Cheese.

Step 2 ADD 2 to 4 tbsp REAL FOOD Yogurt WHIZ.

Step 3 WHIZ till blended. Increase yogurt or cheese for consistency desired.

Step 4 ADD fresh **lemon juice,** and stir in finely chopped **chives** as desired.

CASHEW SPREAD, MAYONNAISE, OR VEGETABLE DRESSING

Step 1   1 c water
½ c roasted cashews
WHIZ in processor or blender till smooth.

Step 2   Cook until thickened.

Step 3   Remove from heat and add:
salt to taste
2½ tbsp fresh lemon juice
½ tsp garlic powder
¼ tsp onion powder
Paprika and **herbs** to taste
STIR and pour into refrigerator jar and CHILL.

AVOCADO DRESSING

1 or 2 soft ripe avocados

WHIZ in food processor or blender till soft and smooth. Stop and push down sides when necessary.

ADD **1 to 2 tbsp lemon juice** and **salt** to taste.

Optional: ½ c orange juice

POUR into refrigerator jar and CHILL, or use at once over green salad.

HOMMUS (*t*)

2 c cooked garbanzos
1 clove garlic
3 tbsp fresh lemon juice

WHIZ in food blender till beans are smooth. A bit of water may be needed for blades to operate. Keep thick. Push down as needed with rubber spatula.

ADD salt to taste, finely **chopped parsley** and **herbs** as desired.

Spread in **Pocket bread** for dressing, or spread over toast.

REAL FOOD YOGURT from Raw Skim Milk (very low fat)

Use: 1 32-oz. straight-edge jar, sterilized!

2 tbsp Yogurt

(Must be acceptable brand containing only l. bulgaricus and s. thermophilus without gelatin or additives). Continental plain is acceptable brand.

4 cups raw skim milk

Step 1 Heat **4 c raw skim milk** slowly until a skin forms on top (161°). Do not boil. COOL to 110°.

Remember, too hot will kill culture; too cold will not allow it to grow.

Step 2 ADD the **2 tbsp Yogurt** to milk, mixing well, and pour immediately into a PREHEATED, hot 32-oz GLASS, straight-edge jar. WORK QUICKLY.

Step 3 WRAP AT ONCE in a warm heavy cloth, or towel. Place inside a WOOL BLANKET that has been shaped into a well in a suitable cardboard box. Place the box (and yogurt) in a warm and draft-free closet for SIX HOURS.

HINT: If left longer, the culture will be aging and will start turning tart. The short, 6-hour incubation period makes for a sweeter yogurt! However, yogurt may be left 12 to 14 hours without harm. REMOVE from wrapping and carefully, without disturbing or shaking the yogurt, transfer to refrigerator and CHILL without stirring.

STORING:

Home yogurt has no agar or commercial thickening agents, so YOGURT MUST BE STIRRED **DAILY** to keep the cultures from dividing. One will tend to go towards the top, the other towards the bottom. To prevent condensation in refrigeration, cover only with cloth or paper towel. As yogurt is stirred daily, the culture will tend to thicken. YES, WILL KEEP FOR WEEKS AND MONTHS IF **STIRRED** DAILY!

LARGE AMOUNTS:

Use straight-edge large-mouth gallon jars.

To ½ GALLON of milk use 4 tbsp or ½ CUP yogurt. To 1 GALLON milk use 8 tbsp or ½ CUP yogurt culture. Keep jars at 110° and **work quickly.**

REAL FOOD YOGURT CHEESE (a very low-fat cheese)

Or...what to do with a batch of yogurt that doesn't firm up or curdle or seems a mistake. It sometimes happens!

Step 1 Measure water needed in large kettle to meet the level of the **yogurt** in the **32 oz jar.** (Use empty 32 oz jar. Push down in kettle with water till right amount is found.) See illustration.

Step 2 Place a 4″ square of aluminum foil under the jar of yogurt and place in kettle of water. (This makes a double boiler.)

Step 3 Slowly heat water and yogurt in the "double boiler" on a medium heat to simmer. Allow the yogurt to bathe in this bath until it falls away from sides of jar, and seems to congeal into a firm form that can be cut with a knife. May take an hour or so.

Step 4 Turn off heat and allow to cool. Remove from the bath and cool while preparing next step.

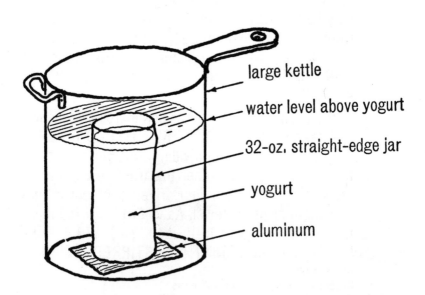

large kettle

water level above yogurt

32-oz. straight-edge jar

yogurt

aluminum

Step 5 Drain away the whey . . . save the curd. Prepare a large pan, place a large sieve over the pan. Dampen a cheesecloth, or handi-wipe, and place over the sieve to hold curd. Carefully cut the curd in the jar and allow it to loosely fall from the jar into the sieve for draining.

Step 6 Forming the curd, or cheese: The curd is the cheese. Let drain until whatever consistency desired. Save whey for soups, bread, etc. For a firm curd, let drain overnight. Hurry process by folding cloth around curd and wring a bit. Taste and use as is. See below.

REAL FOOD YOGURT CHEESE SEASONING SUGGESTIONS

1 c drained curd. Turn into bowl. Use fork or small whip and add any of the following: **dill, caraway,** or **celery seed;** chopped green chili; herbs such as basil, oregano, chives; or, 1 TB mashed pimiento, or add simply salt to taste. SWEETEN the cheese with fruit paste for sweet tooth Real Food.

Cheese Fillings

unseasoned

1. Use Real Food Cheese as is. It contains less than 1 g fat per cup and we know all its contents!

2. Mix ⅔ c yogurt with **1 c HOOP cheese** and WHIZ till smooth. ADD **1 lb dry curd cheese** and contine blending until smooth. Yield 4 c cheese filling.

3. Use **1 c Kefir cheese** as purchased from specialty grocer.

4. Create your own personal combination: i.e., use a **farmer's cheese,** a **very low non-fat cottage cheese,** a **dry curd,** etc. . . . and blend with non-fat or **Real Food yogurt.** Remember to read labels of purchased products!

seasonings . . . use in Real Food Dishes

1. For LASAGNA, add **½ c finely chopped parsley.**

2. For CHEESE, add **4 oz. mashed pimiento.**

3. For DIPS, add **2 tbsp dried onion or garlic chips.**

4. Mix in dashes of **herbs** as for cheeses.

5. SWEET CHEESE FILLING use **fruit paste.**

6. THICKEN with **CHOPPED ONION flakes.**

7. Use cheese filling as base for candies, etc.

8. Use filling as icing for cake or pie!

Milks and Creams

SWEET SESAME CREAM
½ c roasted sesame seeds
¼ c date paste
salt as desired
3 c water

Step 1 Grind seeds till fine in blender or nut grinder.

Step 2 ADD to date paste with half of the water (and salt). WHIZ till smooth.

Step 3 Pour into refrigerator bottle and rinse blender with remaining water and add to milk. REFRIGERATE. Use on cereals, etc.

SESAME MILK
Omit the date paste and salt and use in cooking.

RICE MILK
1 c cooked rice
2 c water
¼ tsp salt (as desired)
¼ to ½ c toasted cashews

Step 1 Dump all into food blender and WHIZ.

Step 2 Pour into refrigerator container, ADD water to make 5 to 6 cups. STIR WELL.

RICE CREAM
Use less ADDITIONAL water in above RICE MILK.

OATMEAL MILK (t)
1 c baby rolled oats
2 c water
vanilla
salt to taste
1 to 2 tbsp date paste

Step 1 WHIZ till smooth. Strain if desired.

Step 2 ADD 2 additional cups water.
OPTIONAL: Add fresh or frozen fruits in the blender till smooth for different tastes. Create!

CASHEW GRAPE CREAM

   1 c white grape juice
   ½ c cashew nuts
   vanilla to taste
   salt as desired

Step 1 WHIZ till smooth.

Step 2 Pour into refrigerator container. Good for dessert topping.

COCONUT MILK

   2 c very hot water
   1 c ground unsweetened coconut
   salt as desired
   MIX coconut and hot water in blender and let stand for a half hour. WHIZ and STRAIN. Refrigerate.

COCONUT CREAM

   ADD **2 tbsp date paste** to above milk for a sweet cream. Refrigerate and use on cereals or in cooking

CASHEW NUT MILK

   1 c raw cashews (or other nut)
   2 c water

Step 1 WHIZ till smooth. ADD 2 more cups water.

Step 2 Refrigerate. Shake well before using.

CASHEW NUT CREAM

   ADD **¼ cup fruit paste** (or other fruit such as apple, banana, papaya, etc.).

SUNFLOWER SEED MILK

SOAK overnight: **1 c shelled sunflower seeds** and 3½ cups of water.

Step 1 WHIZ with 2 cups water until reduced to pulp. ADD remaining water as needed.

Step 2 STRAIN. Pour through fine strainer or thin cloth for a smooth milk. Use the residue in breads or casserole.

BERRY CREAM SHAKE

1½ c cold water
½ c cashews
½ c cooked rice
¼ c date paste
salt as desired

Step 1 WHIZ until smooth.

Step 2 ADD **1 to 2 cups frozen berries** or other frozen fruit. SERVE CHILLED.

CREAM SHAKE (*t*)

1 c cold **fruit juice** or fresh crushed fruit
½ **c date paste** to sweeten
pinch of salt as desired
WHIZ in food blender or processor with metal blade.
ADD additional frozen fruits till thickened as desired.
SERVE.
(Frozen peeled bananas make a good frozen extender.)

Sauces and Toppings FOR VEGETABLES

1. **REAL FOOD clear glaze/sauce:** *t*
   Mix **1 TSP** Arrowroot powder with **½ cup liquid** from the cooked vegetable: (Supplement with cold water or lemon juice). Whiz in blender, or careflly sprinkle the arrowroot into the warm juice while stirring briskly to prevent lumping. Cook only until clear. Either pour the glaze over the vegetables or, stir the vegetables into the glaze.
   GLAZES: CARROTS, MUSHROOMS, ETC.

2. **REAL FOOD VEGETABLE SAUCE:** *t*
   Mix together in blender:
   ¾ c hot water or vegetable juice
   ½ c cooked potato
   ¼ c cooked carrot
   1½ tsp fresh lemon juice

   BLEND until smooth. Pour over vegetables.
   EXCELLENT ON CAULIFLOWER!

3. **REAL FOOD Onion Glaze:** *t*
   ½ c condensed liquid from onion broth
   1 tsp dried onion flakes
   ¼ tsp dried garlic flakes
   pinch of parsley flakes
   season to taste
   1 TSP arrowroot

   Blend until smooth. Put on burner and cook only until clear, stirring constantly. Sauté cooked onions in glaze and let stand keeping warm until served.

4. **REAL FOOD Seasoned Bread Crumbs for topping** *t*
   1 c Real Food or a fat and sugar free bread
   1 tsp mixed spices and herbs
   fresh or dried garlic to taste

   WHIZ all together in processor or blender. Use at once, or dry and store in cool dry place; or freeze until needed.

Fats

"FATS" is a vague, general term for a variety of substances. The following descriptive list is included to underline this fact. The specific meaning of "fats" is of utmost importance in the REAL FOOD diets. These diets discourage use of many fats because of the damage which can occur to our bodies in response to their intake. However, there are natural fats which can aid in the body's maintenance. Particular care then must be taken in response to "fats" in the Real Food Maintenance and Therapeutic diets.

NATURAL FATS:
A "bound fat" that is water soluable, found in unprocessed products "as grown" such as: avocado, nuts, cream, peanut, etc. (These fats are acceptable for the Maintenance Diet.)

*UNNATURAL FATS:
Polyunsaturated and unsaturated fats (both involved in a highly technical process which would take a book to explain).

*REFINED FAT:
12 to 14 ears of fresh corn can be processed in a variety of ways to make only 1 tbsp of a "refined fat" (oily liquid) i.e. corn.

*FREE FATS:
When a natural fat has been taken from or separated away from its original form as in "ear of corn" above, the result is a very concentrated refined fat. It is not water soluable; i.e. grease, oils, lards, etc.

*RANCID FAT:
Any type fat exposed to heat, light, air (oxygen).

*SATURATED FATS:
A solid, i.e. pure lard.

*UNSATURATED FATS:
An oil liquid such as corn oil.

*POLYUNSATURATED FATS:
A thin-pouring oily liquid which is inclined to collect free radicals when exposed to oxygen. (Much damage is then done to the tissues of the body.)

*HYDROGENATED FAT:
Adds hydrogen and thickens; i.e. margarines and shortenings.

*unacceptable to REAL FOOD

Real Food Sweetening

UNREFINED NATURAL FRUIT (as grown)

DATES   **Mejool:** an execeptionally large date with regular size pit, a good buy.

        Honey: small and sweet and usually soft and moist.

        Deglect Noor: medium size and dryer type.

        Khadrawi: a nice sweet type.

        Many other types available ... taste test.

CURRANTS   a mild, non-descriptive flavor

RAISINS   many different kinds; all have different flavors. Taste test.

BANANAS   buy ripe when on sale.

PINEAPPLES   fresh or packed in own juices.

APPLES   all kinds available as well as frozen unsweetened concentrate juice.

GRAPE   bottled unsweetened juices as well as frozen unsweetend concentrate.

All of the above are acceptable to both REAL FOOD Diets

SUGAR — forms of

RAW SUGAR: Made by heating-refining beet or cane juice into crystals and molasses. Raw sugar is illegal in the U.S. because it may contain bacteria, insect parts and dirt from the cane and beets.

TURBINADO SUGAR: A light brown crystal product, is sanitized raw sugar.

BROWN SUGAR: Is white sugar moistened and flavored with molasses. A granular form is also available.

GRANULATED SUGAR: Is white crystals refined to remove all traces of molasses.

CONFECTIONER'S SUGAR: Is powdered white sugar with a tiny percentage of cornstarch added to prevent caking.

SUCROSE: All above which comes from sugar cane and the sugar beet.

LACTOSE: Is a milk sugar.

MALTOSE: Is made with an enzyme that changes starch into malt sugar.

DEXTROSE: Is found in plants, animals and humans and is made commercially by the reaction of sulfuric acid with starch.

FRUCTOSE: Or fruit sugar called LEVULOSE, occurs naturally in fruit and honey, as does ...

LEVULOSE: GLUCOSE. See above.

GLUCOSE: See above.

Dairy Products

Dairy products are not recommended for extensive use in either Therapeutic or Maintenance diets. However, for those who wish to include some limited items, the following list is given with an (*) by the acceptable product. Read labels, and do library research to learn the actual contents of the product you plan to use.

(*) Marks acceptable for Maintenance diet in REAL FOOD

*Raw milk: whole and skim

*Raw whipping cream (will freeze)

*Soft cheeses

*Dry curd cottage cheese

*Hoop cheese

*Plain culture yogurts (no additives)

*Kefir cheese

*Raw non-creamed cottage cheese

*Low-fat cream cheese

*Pasteurized sour cream (no additives)

Non-acceptable to REAL FOOD

Vitamin D "milks"

Canned "milks"

Condensed-sweetened "milks"

Dry "milks"

"half and half"

"whipping cream" (will not freeze)

Hard cheese (i.e. cheddar, etc.)

Butter of all kinds

"yogurts"

Creamed cottage cheeses

Frozen whips or "creams"

Frozen imitations

Ice creams

Ice milks

Gravies, sauces, puddings . . . all products containing "milk"

Sour cream with additives

SEASONING VEGETABLES

There are many different ways to make vegetables taste well seasoned without using too much salt and still avoid harmful substances such as vinegar, black pepper or other spices.

Herbs can be used to enhance the natural flavors of foods. There are no rules to seasoning. Experiment. If you are unfamiliar with an herb, try its effect on various foods by using a small amount at first. If the flavor needs to blend in certain foods, add the flavor at the beginning. If the flavor is to be kept distinct from the food it is used with, add just before serving. Long cooking destroys flavor. Fresh herbs are more desirable in salads. Use 3 times as much fresh than if dried.

The use of lemon juice can perk up the food. Tomato can be used in a similar way, raw and chopped, canned, as sauce or puree. Onion, green pepper, celery, parsley, or garlic will add interesting touches. The addition of chopped nuts or seeds add a delightful flavor, or try a REAL FOOD Glaze.

Asparagus......Lemon juice, lemon thyme, slivered almonds

Beets......Tarragon, sweet basil, thyme, bay leaf, lemon juice

Broccoli......Tarragon, marjoram, oregano, lemon juice, sesame seeds

Brussel sprouts......Sweet basil, dill, savory, thyme

Carrots......Sweet basil, dill, thyme, marjoram, parsley, mint, onion rings, lemon thyme

Cauliflower......Rosemary, savory, dill, parsley, paprika

Cabbage......Caraway, celery seed, savory, dill

Corn......Dill, sweet basil, pimiento, parsley, green pepper

Cucumbers......Lemon thyme, tarragon, sweet basil, savory, dill, lemon juice, paprike

Eggplant......Lemon thyme, sweet basil, thyme, oregano, sage, tomato

Beans (dried)......Sweet basil, oregano, dill, savory, cumin, garlic, parsley, bay leaf, tomato

Green beans......Sweet basil, dill, thyme, marjoram, oregano, savory, tomato, onion, garlic, almonds, mushrooms

Lima beans......Sweet basil, chives, savory

Onions......Lemon thyme, oregano, thyme, sweet basil

Peas......Lemon thyme, sweet basil, mint, savory, oregano, dill, mushrooms, parsley

Potatoes......Lemon thyme, dill, chives, sweet basil, marjoram, savory, parsley

Squash......Sweet basil, dill, oregano, savory, flake yeast

Spinach......Tarragon, thyme, oregano, rosemary

Tomatoes......Rosemary, sweet basil, oregano, dill, garlic, savory, parsley, bay leaf, lemon juice, chives

Green salad dressings......Lemon thyme, sweet basil, parsley, chives, tarragon, lemon juice, thyme, dill, marjoram, oregano, rosemary, savory, mint

Spaghetti sauce......Cumin, sweet basil, oregano, marjoram, onion, garlic, sage

Chili substitute......Spanish onions with cumin

NON-IRRITATING RECOMMENDED HERBS AND SPICES

ANISE SEED* May be used whole or ground on salads, breads or baked fruits. Imparts a mild licorice flavor.

BASIL A natural companion for tomatoes. Use in tomato sauces, vegetable casseroles, soups, stews and any Italian dishes.

BAY LEAF While the leaf itself is not eaten, it imparts flavor and aroma to soups, fish, stews, tomato dishes and fowl. Add one leaf to the pot when you begin cooking and remove before serving.

CARAWAY SEED These seeds add greatly to the flavor of rye bread, sauerkraut, potatoes, soups and stews. Also may be added to cottage cheese for flavoring dips.

CELERY SEED Use as you would celery leaves. Adds delicious flavor to potato salad, soups, stews, fish, tomatoes and salad dressing.

CHIVES A very mild member of the onion family. Used uncooked to flavor sauces, dips and spreads.

CILANTRO Known as Mexican parsley and used widely in Mexican and Chinese cookery. Use sparingly.

CORIANDER May be ground and used in place of cinnamon. Good in vegetable soup (especially pea or lentil) with fish or fowl, bread stuffings and baked fruit.

CUMIN* This spice gives a warm aromatic taste to stews, roasts, meats and root vegetables.

DILL SEED Famous for its use in pickling, salads, fish, soups (especially potato or white bean), and eggs.

FENNEL SEED An herb from the parsley family that imparts a licorice-like flavor. May be used in herb tea, apple pie, fish, Spanish or Italian dishes.

GARLIC A widely-used flavoring agent especially in Italian, Mexican and Middle Eastern dishes. Available as a powder and salt though cloves have the best flavor. There is believed to be an active ingredient in both garlic and onions that helps to lower your serum cholesterol level.

KITCHEN BOUQUET A mixture of herbs, used to flavor soups, stews, and gravies.

MARJORAM From the mint family of France. Used in stuffings, stews, soups, salad dressings, string beans and lima beans.

MINT Imparts an aromatic flavor. Popular for beverages, meats and as a garnish. May be chewed for instant breath refresher.

ONION The most versatile seasoner. May be added to most vegetable or grain dishes. Is often best if first sauteed (can be sauteed in a nonstick pan with a little water if necessary) and then cooked into the main dish.

OREGANO Widely used in seasoning Mexican, Italian, and Greek dishes, as well as tomato sauce and bean dishes.

PAPRIKA (Highly colored Spanish variety) Made from sweet red peppers and used mostly for a garnish rather than a flavoring agent. It makes tomato sauce redder and may be used with eggs, corn, potatoes, goulash, fish and fowl.

PARSLEY Used as a colorful garnish and/or to season soups, salads, stuffings, fish and potatoes. Best for flavor and nutrition if used fresh. May be chewed for an instant breath freshener.

PEPPERMINT (see Mint)

POPPY SEED An Asian herb with a nut-like odor and flavor. Delicious for toppings on breads & rolls.

ROSEMARY A sweet herb that gives a delicate flavor to soups, fish, fowl and salads.

SAFFRON A gourmet's flavoring for fish, soups, rice and curry sauces.

SAGE This herb has a spicy aroma and should be used sparingly in soups, stews, vegetable dishes and bread dressings.

SAVORY Another fragrant herb that lends a delightful flavor to soups, stuffings, cabbage, and salad dressings.

SPEARMINT (see MINT)

SESAME SEED A small seed from the Orient with a nut-like flavor. Used on breads and rolls and vegetable dishes.

TARRAGON A flavoring for salads and many vegetable dishes.

THYME Delicious in bread dressings, soups, meat, and vegetable dishes.

TUMERIC* Used in soups, rice, and other dishes where a rich yellow color is desired. Also good with eggs, corn, potatoes, and salad dressings.

WINTERGREEN (see MINT)

*Some people might find these slightly irritating to their system.